Marwa Shaban

Workplace Hazards In Health Care

Marwa Shaban

Workplace Hazards   In Health Care

Noor Publishing

Imprint

Any brand names and product names mentioned in this book are subject to trademark, brand or patent protection and are trademarks or registered trademarks of their respective holders. The use of brand names, product names, common names, trade names, product descriptions etc. even without a particular marking in this work is in no way to be construed to mean that such names may be regarded as unrestricted in respect of trademark and brand protection legislation and could thus be used by anyone.

Cover image: www.ingimage.com

Publisher:
Noor Publishing
is a trademark of
Dodo Books Indian Ocean Ltd., member of the OmniScriptum S.R.L Publishing group
str. A.Russo 15, of. 61, Chisinau-2068, Republic of Moldova Europe
Printed at: see last page
ISBN: 978-3-330-97091-5

Zugl. / Approved by: Giza,Cairo University,2015

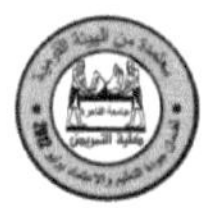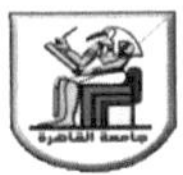

WORKPLACE HAZARDS IN HEALTH CARE

By

Marwa Mamdouh Shaban

Lecturer in Community Health Nursing Department

Faculty of Nursing

Cairo University

2021

WORKPLACE HAZARDS IN HEALTH CARE

Abstract

Background: Dental nurses and dentists were constantly exposed to a number of specific work-related health risk factors which develop and intensify with years. Awareness regarding these work-related health risk factors and implementation of preventive health care measures could provide a safe work environment for all dental nurses and dentists. Aim of the study: To assess the work-related health risk factors among dental nurses and dentists and preventive health care measures applied among dental nurses and dentists. Research design: A descriptive design was utilized. Sample: Convenience sample of 50 dental nurses and 150 dentists were included in the current study. Setting: This study was conducted at the dental clinics at faculty of oral and dental medicine, Al-Kasr Al-Ainy Hospital. Tools of data collection: Three tools were developed, tested for clarity and feasibility: a-Socio-demographic data sheet, b-Work-related health risk factors questionnaire, and c-Structured observational checklist. Results: The most common work risk factors prevailing among dental nurses were emotional exhaustion (82%), low back pain (76%) and latex allergy (62%) and the most common work risk factors prevailing among dentists were percutaneous exposure incident (100%), emotional exhaustion (100%) and low back pain (93.3%). Also, statistically significant negative correlation (r=-0.274, at p = 0.045) between the incidence of chemical health risk factors and application of chemical preventive measures among dental nurses. A statistically significant negative correlation (r=-0.177, at p = 0.030) between the incidences of mechanical health risk factors among dentists and application of mechanical preventive measures. Conclusion: The studied dental nurses and dentists exposed to many work-related health risk factors as latex allergy, percutaneous exposure incidents, low back pain and emotional exhaustion related to inappropriate application of preventive health care measures. Recommendation: Raise awareness of dental nurses and dentists about work-related health risk factors, design and implement health education program for preventive health care measures.

Key words: Work-related risk factors, Preventive Measures, Nurses, Dentists.

Table of Content

LIST OF TABLES

LIST OF ABBREVIATIONS

ADA   American Dental Association

AIDS   Acquired Immune Deficiency Syndrome

BADN   British Association of Dental Nurses

CDC   Centers for Disease Control and Prevention

Db   Decibel

DHCP   Dental Health Care Personnel

FDA   Food and Drug Administration

GAD   Generalized Anxiety Disorder

HAV   Hepatitis A Virus

HBsAg   Hepatitis B Surface Antigen

HBV   Hepatitis B Virus

HCV   Hepatitis C Virus

HIV   Human Immunodeficiency Virus

ICD-10   Tenth Revision of International Classification of Diseases and Related Health
           Problem

MSDS   Material Safety Data Sheet

NIHL   Noise Induced Hearing Loss

NIOSH   National Institute of Occupational Safety and Health

OSHA   Occupational Safety and Health Administration

PCP   Pneumocystis Carini Pneumonia

PEI   Percutaneous Exposure Incidents

PPE   Personal Protective Equipment

PT-NANB   Parenterally Transmitted non-A non-B hepatitis

UV   Ultra Violet

WHO   World Health Organization

CHAPTER I

Introduction

Throughout the world, most adults spent most of their day at work. The work provided a number of benefits as economic, develop new skills, shape the personal identity, and develop the sense of production and value. At the same time people in work faced a variety of risks owing to chemical factors, biological agents, physical factors, mechanical conditions and varied psychosocial factors. In addition to risks, more than 100 occupational diseases had been classified according to the tenth revision of the International Classification of Diseases and Related Health Problems (ICD-10) among workers. Broadly, occupational hazards included respiratory, musculoskeletal, cardiovascular, reproductive, neurotoxic, skin and psychological disorders, hearing loss and cancer (Barrientos & Driscoll, 2012).

Therefore, health care professionals should have knowledge about workforce populations, work-related health risk factors, methods to prevent and control work-related health risk factors to improve health of workers. The work related health risk factors were identified as a chemical, physical, biological or other agent that might cause harm to an exposed person in the workplace and was potentially modifiable. The work of the dental nurses and dentists included a variety of work-related health risk factors, such as working for long hours at a high level of concentration, working in a sedentary state, working with anxious patients, exposure to microbial aerosols generated by high-speed rotary hand pieces and exposure to various chemicals used in clinical dental practice (Fasunloro & Owotade, 2012).

Gupta, Mehta, & Upadhyaya, (2012) categorized the work - related health risk factors among dental nurses and dentists as physical, mechanical, chemical, biological and psychological. Physical health risk factors included eye injuries occurring from projectiles, cuts from sharp instruments, or puncture wounds from needles or other sharp instruments. Such injuries could result in the transmission of serious infectious diseases to the dental nurses and dentists. Also harmful radiation like Non-ionizing radiation (visible light) and (Ultra Violet light) (UV) and ionizing radiation (X-rays) could cause damage to various body cells. Noise and vibration from the hand piece could lead to hearing problems.

Mechanical health risk factors like wrist ache, lower backache, and neck ache could occur due to the need to work in specific working positions using a continuous repetitive motion. Chemical health risk factors could be Inorganic (mercury toxicity), organic (solvents, resins, gases), caustic (formaldehyde, hydrogen peroxide), toxicity from anesthetic gases (nitrous oxide) and latex glove allergy (contact dermatitis). Dental nurses and dentists exposed to biological health risk factors as a result of direct or indirect contact with traumatized tissues, saliva and blood on a daily basis. So that they were at risk of exposure to Hepatitis B Virus (HBV), Hepatitis C Virus (HCV), and HIV (Human Immunodeficiency Virus) and other types of communicable infections. As well as, psychological health risk factors could arise due to stress/excess work load, lack of job satisfaction/insecurity, professional burnout, and medico-legal problems (Kedjarune, Leggat & Smith, 2010).

According to the National Library of Medicine, (2012) the dental nurses and dentists must use preventive health care measures to protect them against the work related injury or illness. The preventive health care measures defined as; the measures taken to prevent diseases or injuries rather than curing them or treating their symptoms. It is also known as the practices that used to protect the workers from work related injury or illness that could be occurring at the workplace setting.

Dental nurse and dentist were responsible for implementing preventive health care measures in clinical practice to reduce the exposure to work-related risk factors, injuries or illness by altering the manner in which a task is performed. For compliance with preventive health care measures; dental nurses and dentists must understand how the health risk factors occurred , what personal protection was needed, when and how to use it correctly, what vaccinations were needed and why, as well as how to keep the practice clean and hygienic, and what to do in the event of an exposure incident such as a skin penetrating injury with a sharp instrument, how to protect yourself from the risks of the chemical disinfectants and how to ergonomically use the instruments and what were the measures used to reduce the work related stress or tension such as effective time management for the work demands and the workloads (Feyer, 2012).

However the prevention of health risk factors in the workplace was central to the practice of occupational health nurse as a profession. The occupational health nurses played an important role in maintaining the health and safety of health care worker through the three level of prevention, primary level of prevention included assessing the work site for risk factors, potential risk factors, reduced risk that could lead to serious injury or disease through initial and periodic mandatory training in the use of Personal Protective Equipment (PPE) and universal precautions, periodic re-evaluation to encourage preventive activity and use of personal protective equipment. Also Immunization review and updated programs, monitoring exposures to infectious disease, maintenance of workers' health records, establishing work restriction programs to prevent transmission of communicable disease, providing educational sessions and literature encouraging work and personal hygiene (World Health Organization [WHO], 2011a).

Buchta & Russi, (2012) the secondary prevention level included developing occupational health and safety strategies by providing nurse direct care through established protocols; risk assessment, health surveillance, environmental health management, risk management and the control of workplace health hazards and could make a useful contribution to the overall management of health and safety at work, with particular emphasis on 'health' risk assessment and management. As well as, in the tertiary prevention level; the occupational health nurse was often the key person in the rehabilitation program who with the manager and the workers complete a risk assessment, devise the rehabilitation program, monitor progress and communicate with the workers, coordinate health care services for the workers from the onset of injury or illness to a safe return to work or an optimal alternative.

Significance of the study

Many studies clarified that dental nurses and dentists reported more frequent and worse health problems than other high risk medical professionals. At Ajman University of Science and Technology described the work-related health risk factors as a study done among dental nurses and dentists in the United Arab of Emirates, 68% from the dental nurses and dentists complained of mechanical health risk factor as a result of musculoskeletal pain, the dental nurses and dentists complained of physical health risk factors included that 42% had percutaneous injury, 53% had eye problems, and 5% had hearing problems followed by 18% complained of chemical health risk factor due to contact dermatitis mostly caused by latex gloves (Al-Ali, Khalid, & Raghad, 2012).

At Damascus university a study done to describe the exposure of dental nurses and dentists in Damascus to some occupational risks and found that 60.7% of dental nurses and dentists complained of chemical health risk factors due to the regular contact with dental amalgam, while 57.9% of dental nurses and dentists complained of mechanical health risk factor related to the backache was the most frequently experienced risks of the subjects and

38.7% of dental nurses and dentists exposed to physical health risks due to the injury from sharp instruments (Ammar, Samer, & Sharif, 2009).

Therefore, this study could contribute greatly to the occupational health nurse through identification of work- related health risk factors as well as the preventive health care measures that could be applied to be in a safe and free hazardous work environment.

Aim of the study

The aim of the study will be two folds:-

- Assess the work-related health risk factors among dental nurses and dentists.

- Assess the preventive health care measures applied among dental nurses and dentists.

Research Questions:

To fulfill the aim of this study, the following research questions will be formulated:

(1)   What are the work-related health risk-factors that prevailing among dental nurses and dentists?

(2)   What are preventive health care measures that are applied by dental nurses and dentists?

CHAPTER II

Review of Literature

The Work-related health risk factors defined as impairments, injuries and illnesses that cause great human suffering and incur high costs, both for those affected and for society as a whole. The work-related health risk factors normally developed over a period of time because of workplace conditions that might include exposure to disease-causing bacteria and viruses or to chemicals and dust. Also, it could be defined as a condition that resulted from exposure in a workplace to a physical, chemical or biological agent which was affecting the normal physiological mechanisms were causing impairment in the health of the worker (Occupational Safety and Health Administration [OSHA], 2013).

In dentistry, the dental nurses and the dentists had more frequent work-related health risk factors than other high risk health professionals. They exposed to various work-related health risk factors like stress, allergic reactions, higher noise levels, radiation, mechanical disorders, and legal hazards. Other work-related health risk factors as interactions with patients, physical strain and financial pressure negatively related to psychological well being of dental professionals. Work-related health risk factors among dental nurses and dentists were categorized as, physical, mechanical, chemical, biological and psychological (Adel & Mustafa, 2012).

<u>Physical work- related health risk factors:-</u>

The physical work - related health risk factors among dental nurses and dentists included eye injuries, percutaneous injuries, exposure to harmful radiation like Non-ionizing radiation (visible and UV light), ionizing radiation (X-rays) and hearing problems as a result of continuous usage of the handpiece that produced a varied level of noise and vibration. Eye injuries during dental practice might have serious and long term effect and sometimes led to loss of vision in one or both eyes, such as direct mechanical trauma often correlate with the severity and type of trauma, and included pain and blurring of vision. Another type of the eye injury was penetrating ocular trauma might lead to serious complications and required extensive surgery. In addition to chemical injuries could result in corneal damage and led to visual impairment and discomfort, which might limit a dental nurses and dentist's future clinical practice (Kanski, 2010).

Albadour & Othman, (2010) described that eye infection were common among dental nurses and dentists that could be caused as a result of contamination of the eye with bodily fluid accidentally such as blood and saliva carried with it several potential risks, both bacterial and viral. Since the surface of the eye was a vital structure, simple contact with an infected substance, for example from a contaminated aerosol, had the potential to cause infection, without the need to be abrased or breached. Also, removal of bacteria laden calculus could cause both physical and microbial infections if projected into the unprotected eye. Of utmost concern was the spread of viral pathogens through aerosols of blood or saliva.

Percutaneous injuries were a frequent problem among dental nurses and dentists, who were among the healthcare professionals the most involved in occupational accidents particularly, needle stick and sharp instrument injuries. This exposure was related to the fact that dental nurses and dentists worked in a limited-access and restricted-visibility field and frequent use sharp devices. Percutaneous Exposure Incident (PEI) was facilitated transmission of blood borne pathogens such as HIV, HCV and HBV (Greenspan & Scully, 2012).

The most common "sharp" injuries among dental nurses and dentists continued to rise from needles and drilling instruments, such as burs. Of concern in needle stick injuries, was the fact that they often occurred while giving injections, when there was usually some residual bodily fluid in the needle from the punctured site. The infection risk after accidents were involving contaminated blood contact depended on various factors, such as: type of exposure, inoculums size, host response, infectious material involved, and the amount of blood (Greenspan & Scully, 2012).

Cheng, Haung & Yen, (2012) described that dental nurses and dentists were known to be a high-risk group for exposure to needle stick injuries, and most dental nurses and dentists experienced at least one needle stick injury during their profession life. There were several reports of occupationally acquired HCV and HIV infection in dental nurses and dentists were following needle stick injury, and reported of HIV transmission to patients from dentists were published during the last two decades. This has raised concerns about compliance with infection-control procedures, which were recommended to protect dental nurses and dentists against blood-borne infections.

The most dental offices and clinics had x-ray machines that were in frequent use, so the dental nurses and dentists were exposed to both ionizing and non-ionizing types of radiations. Ionizing radiation was a well established risk factor for cancer. Also eye irritation, burn, dermatitis and serious injuries could be the associated potential risks from the exposure to the ionizing radiation. Non-ionizing radiation had recently become a concern since the introduction of composites and other resins, in addition to the introduction of lasers in dentistry, which had added another potential hazard to the eye could cause damage to the various structures of the eye, included the retina and the cornea and other body tissues (Chikte, Naidoo, & Yengopal, 2011).

Anyel & Scully, (2011) identified that ionizing radiation from diagnostic radiography machine was the greatest source of radiation hazard in dentistry. Radiographs were essential to dentists for diagnosis, treatment planning, monitoring treatment or lesion development. However, an integral part of radiography was exposure of patients and, potentially dental nurses and dentists to X-rays. The sources of ionizing radiation in the dental clinics were intra-oral, panoramic radiography that was widely used in dentistry and relatively safe, cephalometry was more hazardous as the radiation level was high. No exposure to X-rays could be considered completely free of risk, so the use of radiation by dental nurses and dentists was accompanied by a responsibility to ensure appropriate protection.

Non-ionizing radiation was another source of radiation in dentistry. This has recently become a concern for the use of composites and other resins, next to the use of lasers in dentistry procedures, which had added another potential hazard to the eye and other tissues that might be directly exposed and could cause eye damage, burn and the risk of fire and electrical shock. The effect of laser on the target tissue depended on the wave length, beam power, degree of focus, duration of exposure and distance to target as well as the degree of absorption by the tissue. All lasers should be used with great care and never shown to the eyes, in unintended directions or onto brightly plated instruments which reflect the laser (Samaranayake, 2012).

Isfahan, (2012) identified that dental nurses and dentists were at risk for noise-induced hearing loss. Although hearing loss might not be symptomatic, the first complication and the reason for seeking a hearing evaluation might be tinnitus. Noise is always present during the work of dental nurses and dentists divided into distracting noise and destructive noise. This division resulted from the variety of parameters determining sound hazards and their influence on the human organism. The sources of dental sounds inducing hearing loss that could be diminished were high-speed turbine hand pieces, low-speed handpieces, high-velocity suction, ultrasonic instruments and cleaners, vibrators and other mixing devices, and model trimmers. At least, it should be worth mentioning that air conditioners and office music played too loud.

Noise levels at a given intensity and duration in any environmental situation was a potential health risk-factor. Since the development of new dental instruments and equipment, the potential for auditory problems had been a concern for the dental nurses and dentists. Factors influencing the risk of acoustic trauma are age, physical condition, existing hearing condition of the individual, intensity or loudness (measured in Decibels) (Db) of the equipment, length of exposure, and the time between exposures. The air-driven high-speed handpiece was often identified as a potential noise hazard. Early model handpieces had increased noise levels reported between 80-94 Db at 12 inches and 75-104 Db at six inches, which posed some risk of causing hearing impairment. Currently available models had decibel levels equal to or lower than the standards set by the occupational safety and health act of 90 Db maximum for eight hours of permissible continuous exposure per day (American Dental Association Journal [ADA], 2012).

Studies had been shown the risk of developing Noise Induced Hearing Loss (NIHL) in the dental clinic was minimal. However, dental nurses and dentists should be aware that any potential health risk factors due to noise levels do exist in the dental environment and that everyday noise exposures such as those associated with transportation, power tools, and entertainment produced an additive effect. Hearing loss also increased with years of exposure and in a logarithmic relation to exposure duration. There was no way to undo the damage caused by noise once it has been occurred, so prevention was essential (OSHA, 2013).

<u>Mechanical work-related health risk factors:-</u>

Sartolio & Vercelli, (2012) described that dental nurses and dentists were at a greater risk of work-related mechanical risk-factors than was the general population. It included low back pain, shoulder pain, neck pain and hand/wrist pain. These disorders could result in pain and dysfunction of the neck, back, and hands and fingers. It has been estimated that work-related musculoskeletal injuries occur in 54% to 93% of dental nurses and dentists, with the most frequent injuries were occurring in the spine (neck and back), shoulders, elbows and hands. While specific procedures placed the dentists at increased risk of finger and hand injuries, poor posture was a risk factor with all procedures.

The main risk-factors were responsible for work-related mechanical risk-factors in dental nurses and dentists included repetitive and/or unnatural movements and posture. An increased risk of musculoskeletal injuries and disorders was known to exist in people employed in occupations involving manually repetitive and awkward movements and positions. Finger and hand injuries were more frequent with repetitive demanding movements that additionally involved the application of pressure; in dentistry hand scaling, root planning, and the use of hand files and reamers for endodontic therapy were examples that place the dentists at risk (Morse, Braunea, & Sanders, 2012).

While specific procedures were placed the dentists at increased risk of finger and hand injuries, poor posture was a risk factor with all procedures for both dental nurses and dentists. This was compounded by the requirement to remain in one position for significant lengths of time while performing procedures. Poor postural muscle strength could also lead to forward flexed postures, especially after working for several hours. Stress and time demands could add their toll, with dental nurses and dentists were becoming unaware of poor body position and posture (Melchior, Evanof, & Chastang, 2012).

Mechanical health risk factors (low back pain, shoulder pain, neck pain and hand/wrist pain) were characterized by the presence of discomfort, disability or persistent pain in the joints, muscles, tendons and other soft parts, caused or aggravated by repeated movements and prolonged awkward or forced body postures. Dental nurses and dentists were usually included among the professionals with a higher incidence of musculoskeletal diseases in the course of their professional life. While the occasional backache or neck ache was not a cause for alarm, if regularly feeling of pain or discomfort was ignored, the cumulative physiological damage could lead to an injury or a career-ending disability. Dental nurse and dentist was predisposed to mechanical pain or injury in slightly different areas of the body, depending on his or her tasks and were positioning in relation to the patient include low back pain, shoulder pain and hand/wrist pain as shown in figure (1)

(Valachi, 2010).

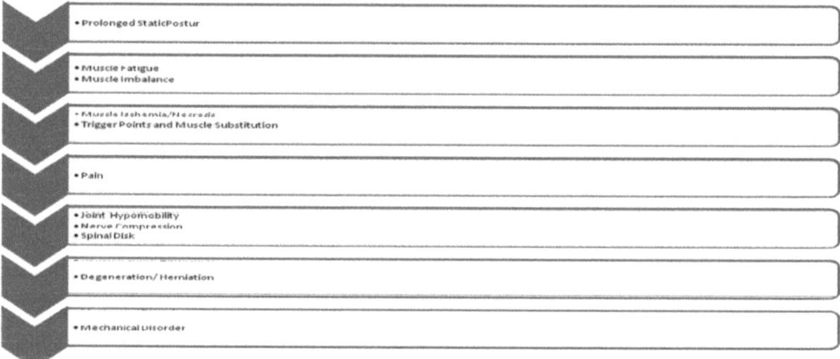

Figure 1. *Flow chart showing how prolonged static postures can progress to pain or mechanical disorder. (Adopted from: Valachi 2010. Mechanisms leading to musculoskeletal disorders in dentistry. The (ADA) Journal. pp 1346).*

At work, the dental nurse and dentist worked in a strained posture (both while standing and sitting close to a patient), which eventually led to overstress of the spine and limbs. This refers to the 37.7% of the work time. The overstress produced a negative effect on the musculoskeletal system and the peripheral nervous system; above all, it affected the peripheral nerves of the upper limbs and the neck nerve roots. Spine degeneration led to back pain syndromes which were reported frequently in dental nurses and dentists. Neck discopathy resulted in cervical pains or cervico-acromial pains, which were particularly common among dentists. The posture which the dentist assumed at work with the neck bent and twisted, an arm abducted, repetitive and precise movements of the hand, were a frequent cause of the neck syndrome and of pain within the shoulder and upper extremities (Jabbar, 2012).

Al-Eisa, (2011) found that the risk for low-back pain was associated with work undertaken for prolonged periods of time in a seated position. Continual seating for a prolonged period resulted in activation of the upper and lower erector spinae muscles, and with significantly greater low-back compressive was loading in the lumbar spine region than exists when standing. In addition, pelvic asymmetry could result in asymmetric trunk movement when was working in a seated position, and that this resulted in significant differences in lower-back pain, proposing that the asymmetric working movements were compensatory and placed the lumbar spine under significantly higher stress.

Lumbar and lumbosacral discopathy arouse pain in the loins and the lower back radiating to the lower extremities, more often right than left. This could be explained by a greater stress on the right side of the body when the dental nurse and dentist worked with a sitting patient. The dental nurse, dentist made constant monotonous movements, which stressed the wrist and elbow joints. Also of consequence were mechanical vibrations which were produced by some dental equipment like ultrasonic scalers and handpieces and were transmitted to the hands and arms. In addition, the extensive use of hand tools in dentistry work could cause a chronic extrinsic compression of the nerves in the hand, and therefore might cause an entrapment of digital nerves. Whatever the cause of the symptoms, neurological disturbances were potentially serious in an occupation in which precise hand movements were necessary (Dawson, Hallet, & Millinder, 2011).

The median nerve and cubital nerve defects were seen in a number of dentists. An early syndrome of a defected median nerve shows in acroparasthesiea. A consequence of the defected median nerve in the carpal nerve was the so-called tunnel syndrome. Its early phase was dominated by paroxysmal parasthesia of the thumb and the index finger, which occurred almost without exception at night and which was accompanied by sensomotor disorders of the thumb and the index finger. Operations were carried out during extractions stress not only the elbow joint and the wrist joint, but might result in chronic tendon sheath inflammation. The long-term effect of all those adverse circumstances occurring in the work of the dentists might lead to diseases described as cumulative trauma disorders (Ostrem, 2011).

<u>Chemical work-related health risk factors:-</u>

Dental nurses and dentists exposed to many of the chemical risk factors included dermatoses, latex glove allergy, mercury toxicity, risks from prolonged usage of chemical disinfectant as: formaldehyde, hydrogen peroxide and other chemical disinfectants. The work-related dermatoses associated with other dental products might be more common. These conditions might be found in more than one-quarter of dental and medical personnel. Dental nurses and dentists should be aware of common chemical allergens, symptoms of allergic contact dermatitis and the appropriate treatment of work- related skin disease. Allergic dental nurses and dentists must be learning to avoid the products that contained the allergen and eliminated or minimized the potential routes of exposure. All dental chemicals that were able to induce allergic reactions and irritation should be handled with sufficient precautions in every dental office (Depaola, Rodgers, & Hamann, 2010).

An intrinsic part of dental nurses and dentist's protective equipment included gloves and mask. Latex gloves had been worn routinely in the dental profession for more than two decades and were the basis of good infection control strategies. However, the residual or integral chemical components posed a potential health risk factor to some dental nurses and dentists. Gloves dusted with cornstarch powder were most often used. The gloves and mask formed an inbuilt barrier against most pathogens, and as recently proven, they also constituted a very good barrier against viruses, provided that the gloves and mask were intact. However, they might produce allergic reactions primarily in those persons who use rubber products on a regular basis and dental nurses and dentists were falling in this category (Hamann, 2012).

The most important risk factor of immediate allergies was frequent exposure to latex products. Sensitization might occur through inhalation of airborne powder or through the skin. The inhaled glove powder was capable of inducing type 1 hypersensitivity responses, but the most common type of allergic reaction was the delayed hypersensitivity or allergic contact dermatitis. The clinical symptoms of latex allergies included: urticaria, conjunctivitis accompanied by lacrimation and swelling of eyelids, mucous rhinitis, bronchial asthma and anaphylactic shock. Cornstarch or the so called absorbable dusting powder also played an important role in latex allergies, manifesting itself in the reaction on the part of the airway. This powder was not biologically neutral, as was previously thought. It was allergenic and taken part in immediate allergic reactions (Charpin & Vervolet, 2011).

However, Tosic, (2011) reported that the most frequent allergy complained in dental practices was probably sensitivity to latex. Powdered latex gloves were mentioned to cause an allergic reaction, although dental nurses and dentists with an allergic profile complained that all latex gloves caused irritation. The powder in latex gloves itself was not the allergen. It only provided binding sites for latex protein, and aided in carrying the protein into the skin. It had also been reported that airborne powder particles could cause asthmatic allergic reactions or even anaphylaxis. Dental nurses and dentists should also note that latex was presented in the other PPE, e.g. masks, eyewear, and clinical gowns. These items had been linked to adverse skin and mucous membrane reactions.

There were three basic categories of adverse latex gloves allergy associated conditions as identified in Table (1): Delayed hypersensitivity or contact dermatitis (type IV) and irritant contact dermatitis (non immune) as shown in Figure (2), immediate hypersensitivity (type I) as shown in Figure (3). The first type of latex allergy (type I) Immediate hypersensitivity was characterized by urticaria, bronchospasm and anaphylaxis. The fourth type of latex allergy (type IV hypersensitivity) was the least common but the worst type of reaction as shown in Figure (4); it was characterized by popular, pruritic rash, vesicles and blisters. The irritant contact dermatitis (non immune) was the most common among health care workers, especially dental nurses and dentists as a result of the daily working with gloves and repetitive hand washing; it's characterized by dry, cracked and irritated skin. Sufferers from latex allergy should rather use vinyl or nitril gloves, while it was advisable for severe sufferers to work with latex-free environment (Tosic, 2011).

Table 1

Show reactions to latex products. (Adopted from: Reddy 2009. Latex Allergy.American Family Physician Journal; 6,1415.)

Type of reaction	Symptoms	Cause	Time of onset
Immediate hypersensitivity (type I)	Urticaria (local or generalized), Nausea, vomiting, faintness, rhinitis, conjunctivitis, bronchospasm, anaphylactic shock	Latex	Immediate (within minutes)
Delayed hypersensitivity or contact dermatitis (type IV)	Papular, pruritic rash; vesicles; blisters	Chemicals in latex	Delayed (several hours to 48 hours after contact)
Irritant contact dermatitis (non immune)	Dry, cracked, irritated skin	Chemicals in latex or hand washing	Gradual (over several days)

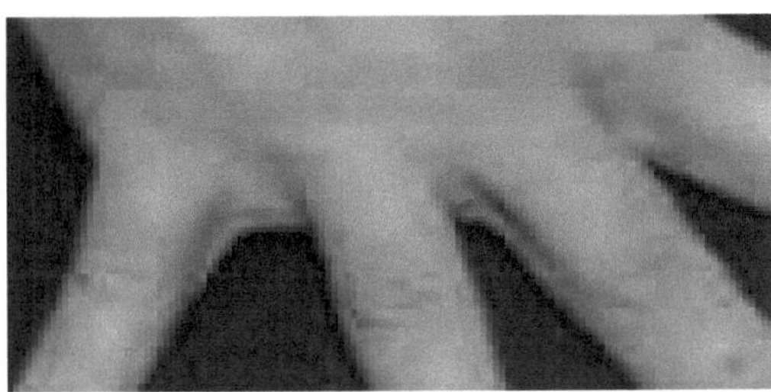

Figure 2. *Irritant contact dermatitis (non immune). (Adopted from Pollart 2009. Latex Allergy .American Family Physician Journal;3,1413).*

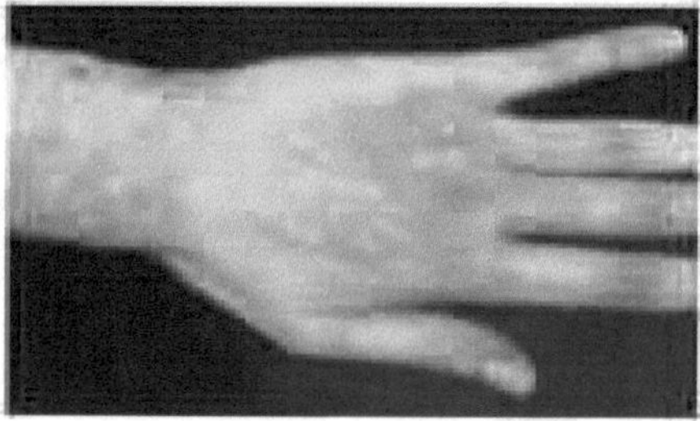

Figure 3. *Immediate hypersensitivity (type I). (Adopted from: Reddy 2009. Latex Allergy .American Family Physician Journal;6,1415).*

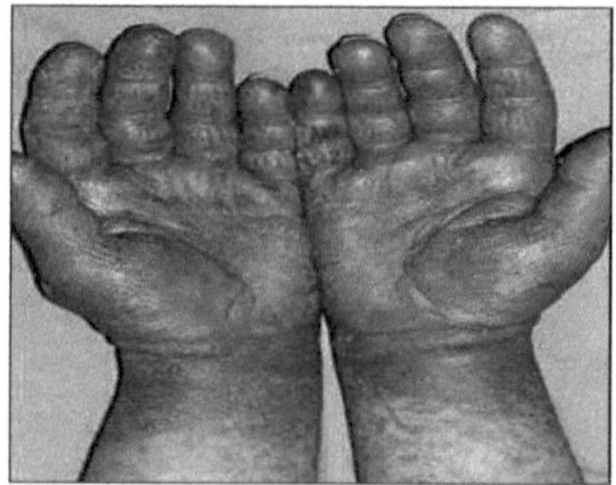

Figure 4. *Type IV delayed hypersensitivity allergy. (Adopted from: Greer 2009.Latex Allergy .American Family Physician Journal;13,1414).*

Dental materials based on methacrylate, its polymer and polyelectrolytes; seemed to be a major cause of contact dermatitis in dental nurses and dentists. Dental nurses and dentists used a variety of different polymer materials. The setting of restorative materials and adhesives was initiated chemically by mixing two components or by visible light. In both cases, polymerization was incomplete and monomers not reacted were released. These free monomers might cause a wide range of adverse health effects such as irritation to skin, eyes or mucous membranes, allergic dermatitis, asthma and parasesthesia in the fingers. Additionally, disturbances of the central nervous system such as headache, pain in the extremities, nausea, loss of appetite, fatigue, sleep disturbances, irritability, loss of memory, and changes in blood parameters might also be noted (Tosic, 2011).

There was also some concern about amalgam safety, included the tenuous hypothesized link between amalgam restorations and specific diseases. Elemental mercury was absorbed through direct skin contact or inhalation, thus it might cause cytogenetic damage and higher blood mercury levels. A lack of evidence to suggest a detrimental health outcome in dentists who were occupationally exposed to higher levels of mercury and were known to have higher levels of mercury in their blood, provided a trend concerning the safety of amalgam (Tosic, 2011).

Although amalgam contained mercury was no longer as widely used as it once was, it was nevertheless frequently encountered in dental procedures and remained a hazard for dental nurses and dentists. Amalgam or "silver filling" contained a mixture of metals such as silver, copper and tin, in addition to mercury, which chemically bind these components to form a hard, stable and relatively safe substance. The greatest exposure to dental nurses and dentists came from handling amalgam for restoration, although storage and disposal of amalgam and amalgam capsules also represented important sources of exposure (Martin & Naleway, 2011).

Lindbohm, (2014) found that chemical disinfectants were a major chemical risk-factor among dental nurses and dentists. Chemical disinfectants were being used in the dental practice to decontaminate hands, instruments and surfaces. Disinfectants that killed germs, viruses, and fungal spores often contain aldehydes (especially formaldehyde and glutaraldehyde) or phenol. Aldehydes were well known for their sensitizing potential and their inhalation toxicity. Exposure to aldehydes at low doses on a continuous basis might lead to chronic toxic effects, the symptoms of which were mostly unspecific (nausea, impairment of the memory, motivation, reactivity or dexterity). Even less toxic alcoholic compounds, such as ethanol, isopropanol, and n-propanol, could cause irritation of the respiratory tracts and the mucous membranes. An unpleasant disinfectant odor had been often the only sign that unhealthy air pollutants were present.

Formaldehyde was one of the chemical agents routinely used in the clinical set up mainly for disinfection of operatory area. Liquid and vapor forms of formaldehyde might cause severe abdominal pain, nausea, vomiting and eye irritation. Inhalation exposure to formaldehyde had also been identified as a potential cause of asthma or asthma-like symptoms. Formaldehyde was a primary skin sensitizing agent and had been associated with both contact dermatitis (Type IV allergy) and anaphylactic reactions (Type I allergy). Inhalation exposure could contribute to the manifestation of allergic contact dermatitis. Occupational Safety measures should be followed to minimize the side effects due to chemical agents (Lyapena, Yaneva, Tzycova, & Garova, 2012).

<u>Biological work-related health risk factors:-</u>

Babaji, Samadi, Jaiswal, & Bansal, (2011) identified that the dental nurses and dentists were at high risk for the biological health risk factors that were constituted by infectious agents of human origin and included viruses, bacteria and fungi. Transmissible diseases currently of greatest concern to the dental nurses and dentists were HCV, HBV, HIV and other upper respiratory diseases or infection. Dental nurses and dentist could become infected either directly or indirectly, i.e. by a cut or wound, needle stick injury, aerosols of saliva and gingival fluid. The following were the main entry points of infection: epidermis of hands, oral epithelium, nasal epithelium, the epithelium of the upper airways, bronchial tubes, alveoli and conjunctival epithelium. In order to overcome the infection spread, a thorough knowledge about the infection, mode of transmission and safety measures was necessary.

Generally, dental nurses and dentists were at far greater risk of exposure to blood borne pathogens such as (HBV, HCV, and HIV) than to, transmitting any of these to the patient, as shown in figure (5). The transmission mode for such exposures primarily due to cut from sharp and needle stick injuries. Manipulations without barrier precautions also increased the risk of infection. Dental nurses and dentists routinely worked in an environment where there was a frequent spatter of blood and bloody saliva and where there was the potential for percutaneous sharps exposure while handling numerous dental instruments. Dental nurses and dentists often work with syringe needles and sharp instrument with a little visualization of the treatment field (Ammon, Reichart, Pauli, & Petersen, 2010).

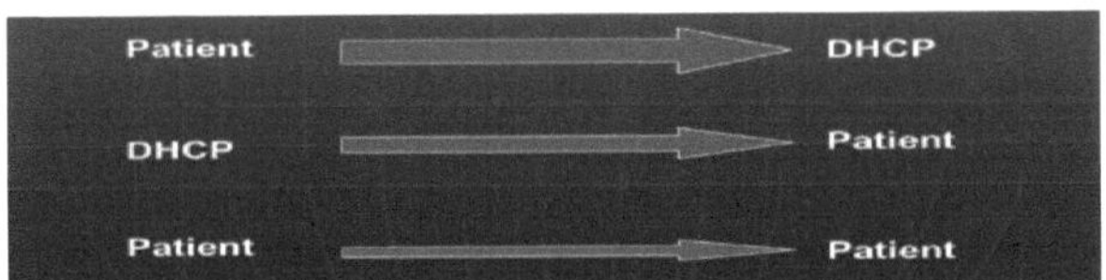

Figure 5. *Potential routes of transmission of blood borne pathogens among dental health care workers. (Adopted from: Saleh 2010. Knowledge, Attitude and Practice Toward blood borne diseases among Dental Health Care Personnel (DHCP) thesis).*

Hepatitis B infection was one of the major diseases of mankind and was a serious global public health problem. It was caused by HBV. The first recorded cases of hepatitis B, formerly called serum hepatitis, were thought to be those that followed the administration of smallpox vaccine was containing human lymph of shipyard workers in Germany in 1883. In the early and middle parts of this century, serum hepatitis was repeatedly observed following the use of contaminated needles and syringes. The role of blood as a vehicle for virus transmission was further emphasized in 1943, when Beeson described jaundice among seven recipients of blood transfusions (WHO, 2010b).

Australia antigen, later called hepatitis B surface antigen (HBsAg), was first discovered in 1963 by Baruch and his colleagues who identified a protein (the Australia antigen) that reacted to antibodies from patients with hemophilia and leukemia. The association of this protein with hepatitis B was discovered three years later by several investigators. The Dane particle (complete hepatitis B virion) was identified in 1970. Identification of serologic markers for HBV infection followed, which helped to clarify the natural history of the disease. Ultimately, HBsAg was prepared in quantity and now comprised the immunogen in highly effective vaccines for the prevention of HBV infection. Hepatitis B had also been called type B hepatitis, serum hepatitis, and homologous serum jaundice (WHO, 2010b).

The dental care environment was a major source of viral transmission. There were many reports of HBV infections acquired through the dental equipment and needle stick injuries. Some medical specialties were associated with greater risk of transmission of HBV as dentistry and surgery. Needle stick injury from an infected needle could result in transmission of HBV in 12% of cases. Health workers were at particular risk of developing the infection. Another common mode of transmission occurred through reuse of contaminated sharp instruments, acupuncture, ear piercing, circumcision and scarification especially in areas of intermediate prevalence of infection (Houivs, 2010).

In dental care settings microorganisms could be transmitted through direct contact with blood, oral fluids, or other patient materials. Indirect contact with contaminated objects (e.g., instruments, equipment, or environmental surfaces) contact of conjunctival, nasal, or oral mucosa with droplets (e.g., spatter) was containing microorganisms generated from an infected person and propelled a short distance (e.g., by coughing, sneezing, or talking) inhalation of airborne microorganisms that could remain suspended in the air for long periods (Fariba &Younai, 2010).

For many of these exposures, transmission of HBV was very plausible because of contamination with blood and saliva. It had been shown that both infectious viruses and HBsAg particles were present in saliva; however, the number of infectious viruses was very low even in HBsAg-positive blood. Generally, percutaneous injuries with sharp instruments such as cutting instruments and anesthetic needles were the most common source of work-related exposures in dentistry. A survey of dental nurses and dentists by the American Dental Association showed that dental nurses and dentists experienced an average of 3.2 injuries per year (Center for Disease Control and Prevention [CDC], 2010a).

Hepatitis C infection was a major global public health problem. It is caused by HCV. The discovery of HCV started in 1975 by the first demonstration that most cases of transfusion-associated hepatitis was caused by neither Hepatitis A Virus (HAV) nor HBV, the only two known human hepatitis viruses at that time, this new form of the disease was called non-A non-B hepatitis and the presumed etiologic agent was non-A non-B hepatitis virus. In 1989, the virus responsible for most transfusion-associated non-A non-B hepatitis was identified, cloned, and named hepatitis C virus. Hepatitis C was also called type C hepatitis, Parenterally Transmitted non-A non-B hepatitis (PT-NANB), non-B transfusion–associated hepatitis, and post transfusion non-A non-B hepatitis (WHO, 2010c).

Work-related exposures of dental nurses and dentists to HCV infection were no greater than the general population, averaging 1% to 2%. The average incidence of anti-HCV seroconversion after accidental percutaneous exposure from an HCV-positive source was 1.8% with one study indicating that transmission occurred only from hollow-bore needles compared with other sharps. Transmission rarely occurred from mucous membrane exposures to blood, and no transmission in dental nurses and dentists had been documented from intact skin exposures to blood (CDC, 2010a).

Data were limited on survival of HCV in the environment. In contrast to HBV, the epidemiological data for HCV suggested that environmental contamination with blood containing HCV was not a significant risk for transmission in health care settings with the possible exception of the hemodialysis setting where HCV transmission related to environmental contamination and poor infection-control practices had been implicated. The risk of transmission from exposure to fluids or tissues other than HCV infected blood (CDC, 2010a).

Acquired Immune Deficiency Syndrome (AIDS) was the most severe consequence of infection with the HIV. It was invariably fatal. AIDS apparently first appeared in 1979, and was brought to the attention of the medical community in 1981. Acquired means caught as opposed to inherited, Immune deficiency implied poor body defense mechanisms against infections, and Syndrome was a group of illnesses which help to identify a particular disease – in this case AIDS. The first report of AIDS came from the center for disease control in Atlanta, Georgia, in the United States which described the cases of 5 young previously healthy homosexuals who had been treated in Los Angeles hospitals for a rare infection of the lungs – Pneumocystis Carini Pneumonia (PCP) (Fauci & Lane, 2010).

In dental care settings, the HIV virus could be transmitted from blood and saliva through needles and sharps, from direct contact through touching or exposing non-intact skin to infective oral lesions, infected tissue surfaces or infected fluids, from inhalation of aerosols or droplets were containing pathogens while were using handpieces and scalers or droplet nucleii from coughing, from indirect contact through fomites by touching contaminated inmate surfaces in the dental treatment room or operatory. In Egypt, the work-related exposure to HIV was mostly due to exposure to needle stick injuries. In a study done in Egypt, out of 1485 health care workers, 529 (35.6%) were exposed to at least 1 needle stick injury during a period of 3 months with an estimated annual number of 4.9 needle sticks per worker. The most common behavior associated with needle stick injures was 2-handed recapping (Talaat *et al*, 2010).

The risks from work-related transmission of HIV had been described; risks varied with the type and severity of exposure. In prospective studies of dental nurses and dentists the average risk for HIV transmission after a percutaneous exposure to HIV infected blood had been estimated to be approximately 0.3% and after a mucous membrane exposure, approximately 0.09%. Although episodes of HIV transmission after non intact skin exposure had been documented, the average risk of transmission by this route had not been precisely quantified, but estimated to be less than the risk for mucous membrane exposures. The risk for transmission after exposures to fluid or tissues other than HIV–infected blood also had not been quantified, but was probably considerably lower than for blood exposures (Bell, 2010).

<u>Psychological work-related health risk factors:-</u>

Not only physical impairments affected dental nurses and dentist's health. Job-related psychological disorders also contributed greatly. Factors that affected dental nurses and dentist's psychological status could be job-related stress, tension, depression, emotional exhaustion (burnout) and depersonalization. Many clinical situations produced stress to dental nurses and dentists and these included, procedures connected with anaesthetization of patients, overcoming of pain and fear, unanticipated emergency situations in which a patient's life was in danger, or procedures with hesitant prognosis. Unskillful planning of a treatment might be a source of disappointment and pain associated with failed both to a dentist and a patient (Isfahan, 2012).

Dental nurses and dentists encountered numerous sources of professional stress, beginning in the dental clinic. Stress could be defined as the biological reaction to any adverse internal or external stimulus, physical, mental or emotional those tend to disturb the organism's homeostasis. Dental nurses and dentists perceived dentistry as being more stressful than other occupations. Coping with difficult or uncooperative patients, over workload, the constant drive for technical perfection, underuse of skills, low self-esteem and challenging environment were important factors contributing to stress among dental nurses and dentists (Dunlap & Stewart, 2011).

Stress might produce "burnout". It was a syndrome of emotional exhaustion, depersonalization and reduced personal accomplishment, a particular type of job-related stress reaction. It was a response to the chronic emotional strain of dealing extensively with other human beings, particularly when they were troubled or having problems. The values of burnout and its constituents among dental nurses and dentists were amazingly high. Recent findings suggested that burnout had features of maladaptive coping in the short term, but was, paradoxically, protective in the longer term. Dental nurses and dentists were prone to burnout due to the nature of their work, but might be able to prevent it if they could recognize the burnout process and take regular holiday breaks (Puriene, 2011).

Rada & Johnson, (2011) defined burn out as: "A syndrome of emotional exhaustion, depersonalization and reduced personal accomplishment that could occur among individuals who do people work of some kind." Burnout was best described as a gradual erosion of the person. Prolonged experience of burn out might lead to depression,

so early recognition of the symptom was important. In a study of three dental specialties'
by Humphris, (2011) reported that general dentists and Oral surgeons had the highest
levels of burnout and that orthodontists had the lowest levels of burnout.

Depression might be a consequence of prolonged experience of burnout. There
was a relationship between emotional load and volume of patients treated.
Depersonalization levels decreased with age and it could be due to a number of factors –
socialization skills, were increasing with age, a slowing of the pace of work which allows
more personal contact, or the establishment of personal relationships with patients over
time. Older dentists worked fewer hours, with a larger impact of age seen among men.
Emotional support might be gained from co-workers that were why the numbers of burnout
syndrome might decrease in the larger practice groups. Conversely, a particular
characteristic of private practice was the high level of control. It allowed dentists to have
control over their working conditions a factor which was reported to help reduce stress
levels (Osborne & Cruocher, 2011).

Rada & Johnson, (2011) explained that dental nurses and dentists might be
experiencing anxiety disorders and depression during their work. Anxiety disorders were
chronic and relentless and could grow progressively worse if not treated. Two common and
potentially overlapping anxiety disorders were panic disorder and Generalized Anxiety
Disorder (GAD). In panic disorder, feelings of extreme fear and dread strike unexpectedly
and repeatedly for no apparent reason they were accompanied by intense physical
symptoms like feeling sweaty, weak, faint, dizzy, flushed or chilled; having nausea, chest
pain, smothering sensations, or a tingly or numb feeling in the hands. GAD was
characterized by chronic exaggerated worry and tension, even though little or nothing had
provoked it.

Depressive disorder often had been occurred with anxiety disorders and substance abuse. Major depression was an illness that involved the body, mood and thoughts. It affected the way people eat, sleep, feel about themselves and thought about things. Studies had been indicated that both anxiety and depressive disorders were observed frequently in both the dental nurses and dentist. Depression might be a consequence of prolonged experience of burnout and it was considered as a sign of the psychological impairment resulted from job related stress in dental practice (Humphris, 2011).

<u>Preventive health care measures:-</u>

The National Library of Medicine, (2012) defined the preventive health care measures as the measures taken to prevent diseases or injuries rather than curing them or treating their symptoms. It was also known as the practices that used to protect the workers from work related injury or illness that could be occurring at the workplace setting. All health care workers should have access to preventive health care measures guidelines that advice about the management of the various work related risk factors or injuries. It should include clear written instructions on the appropriate action to take in the event of any of the work risk factors done such as in the event of a needle stick injury, other blood or body substance exposures, and spillage of chemical disinfectant. All health care workers were encouraged to report occupational exposures immediately and all testing procedures and follow-up treatment should be fully documented.

The preventive health care measures were important in the practice of dentistry because dental nurses and dentists were exposed to a wide variety of health risk factors include physical, mechanical, chemical, biological and psychological. The international literature focused mostly on infection control and proper handling of potentially infected materials to prevent the transmission of microorganisms might include HBV, HCV, HIV also there was importance for the dental nurses and dentists to apply preventive health care measures to protect them against the risk of radiation, occurrence of eye injury, skin penetrating injury with a sharp instrument, the risks of the chemical disinfectants and how to ergonomically use the instruments and what are the measures used to reduce the work related stress or tension such as effective time management for the work demands and the workloads (CDC, 2010b).

<u>Preventive health care measures for the physical work-related health risk factors:-</u>

Kohn *et al*, (2010) explained the following measures for eye safety include protective eyewear and face shields. The protective eyewear must be worn during procedures that involved splash and spatter of saliva and blood. Eyewear protected the eyes from damage and microbes which could be transmitted through the conjunctiva. The face shields served as barriers to protect the mucous membranes of the eye, nose, and mouth from spatter. Eyewear and face shields should be washed with an appropriate cleaning agent and when visibly soiled, disinfected between patients.

The preventive health care measures that used to eliminate or reduce percutaneous exposure incidents by using and caring of sharp instruments and needles. Sharp items (e.g., needles, scalpel blades, wires) contaminated with patient blood and saliva should be considered as potentially infective and handled with care to prevent injuries. Used needles should never be recapped or manipulated utilizing two hands. If needles had to be recapped either a one–handed "scoop" technique as shown in the figure (6) or a mechanical device designed for holding the needle sheath should be employed as shown in the figure (7). Used disposable syringes and needles, scalpel blades, and other sharp items should be placed in an appropriate puncture-resistant container located as close as possible to the area in which the items were used. Needles should never be bent, break or cut before disposal (CDC, 2010b).

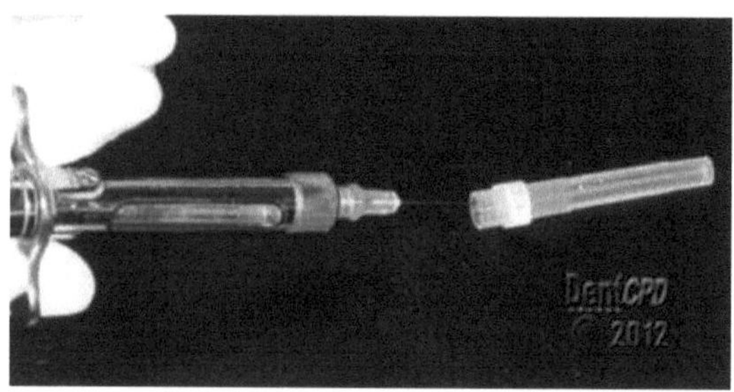

Figure 6. *One-hand technique to recap the needle. (Adopted from: Dickinison 2012 .Sterilization and cross-infection control in the dental practice. Dental CPD journal. pp14).*

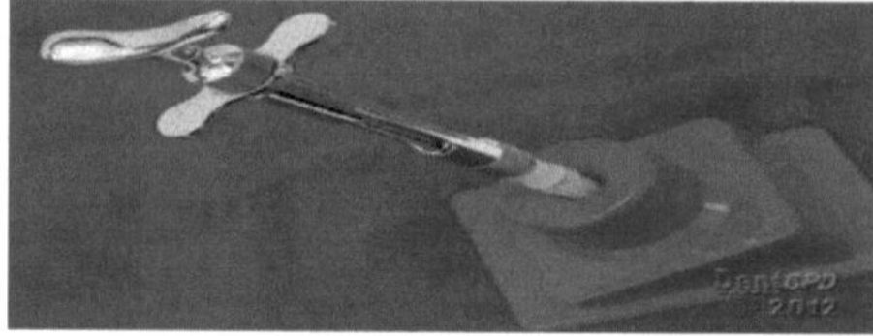

Figure 7. *Mechanical means for holding the needle. (Adopted from: Dickinson 2012 .Sterilization and cross-infection control in the dental practice. Dental CPD journal. pp14).*

In addition to protecting the dental nurses and dentists from percutaneous exposure incidents by disposal of waste materials, included disposable needles, scalpels, or other sharp items should be placed intact into puncture resistant containers before disposal. Solid waste contaminated with blood or other body fluids should be placed in a color–coded or labeled container that prevented leakage (e.g., Biohazard bag) and then disposed safely. Blood, suctioned fluid, or other liquid waste might be poured carefully into a drain connected to a sanitary sewer system (CDC, 2010b).

Also the exposure to both ionizing and non-ionizing radiation might occur in dental practice. Radiographies equipment was common place in dental clinics and radiographs were an integral part of the clinical assessment. As such, it was important that good radiation practice to protect both dental patient and staff. Dental nurses and dentists should take steps to protect themselves during exposures by standing behind protective barriers, use of radiation monitoring badges, wearing of lead apron and regular equipment checks. They should use heat–tolerant or disposable intra- oral devices whenever possible (e.g., film holding as shown in the figure (8) and positioning devices). Clean and heat–sterilize heat–tolerant devices between patients, transport and handle exposed radiographs in an aseptic manner to prevent contamination of developing equipment (Kedjarune *et al*, 2010).

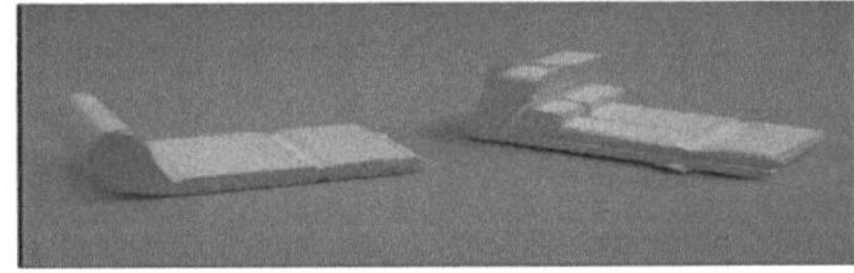

Figure 8. *Disposable film holder. (Adopted from: Dickinson 2012 .Sterilization and cross-infection control in the dental practice. Dental CPD journal. pp20).*

Non-ionizing radiation had become an increasing concern among dental nurses and dentists with the use of the use of lasers in dentistry procedures, ultraviolet and blue light to cure or polymerize various dental materials, especially composite resin, bonding agents and sealants. Safety shields and glasses have been shown to be protective in this regard when used correctly. Other PPE as shown in the figure (9) (e.g., masks, eyewear, and protective clothing) was required when splatter or splash was anticipated (Isfahan, 2012).

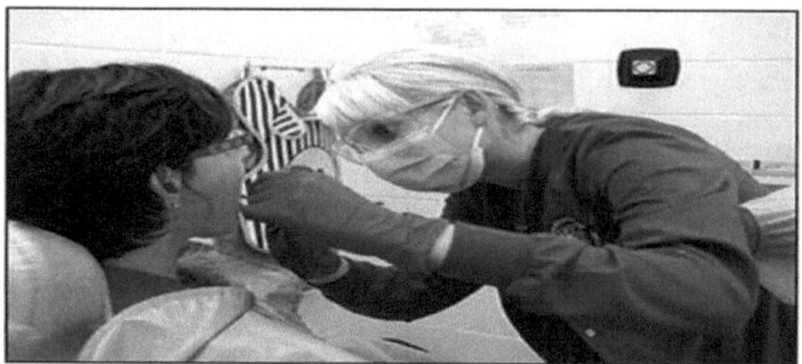

Figure 9. *Personal Protective Equipment (PPE). (Adopted from: Dickinson 2012. Sterilization and cross-infection control in the dental practice. Dental CPD journal. pp20).*

The National Institute of Occupational Safety and Health, (NIOSH, 2012) has been set the following safety standard recommendations for the dental nurses and dentists to protect them from the hearing problems that induced from handpieces and vibration of machines during any dental procedures, the handpieces should be adjusted to below 85 Db for eight-hour exposure, an audiometric test should be taken at the start of employment and every sixth year thereafter, with checkup audiograms every two years, when the noise intensity was above the recommended level, engineering controls should be used to reduce exposure, PPE should be utilized by individuals exposed to noise above the recommended level and are required for noise exceeding 115 Db. Also dental nurses and dentists who exposed to noise should be informed of risks, symptoms, and precautions.

Preventive health care measures for the mechanical work-related health risk factors:-

Valachi B., & Valachi K., (2013) explained the preventive health care measures for mechanical health risk factors as working ergonomically help prevent work-related injuries. The dental nurses and dentists must be optimized his or her working environment to help eliminate awkward postures, physical wear and tear, and fatigue; he or she must position the body in order to clearly visualize the operative site without unnatural body positioning. Dental chairs, stools, magnification devices, visualization aids and dental equipment had all helped improve ergonomics for working dental nurses and dentists. Sitting in an appropriate chair, using magnification for visualization and selecting ergonomic equipment were all essential for the health of dentists. Attention must be given to changing destructive postural habits and selecting equipment conducive to good posture.

The most important measure to prevent the occurrence of low back pain was the appropriate selection of the dental stool or chair. Posture varied depending on the dental stool selected, so careful selection was crucial. The dental stool must fit correctly; it must offer neutral back, neck and shoulder support for optimal posture; must be at the correct height and tilt; and most offer optional arm and elbow support. One size didn't not fit all there were wide variations in dentists' heights and body shapes, and the stool must fit the dentists for whom it is intended. An incorrectly fitting chair may exacerbate rather than reduce the risk of work-related musculoskeletal injuries. Important design considerations included the height of the stool's cylinder, the depth of the stool and the style and presence of armrests (El-Eisa, Egan, Deluzio, & Wassersug, 2008).

Dental stools might have a horizontal, tilting seat as appeared in the figure (10) or saddle-style seat as appeared in the figure (11). Horizontal seats could result in posterior rotation of the pelvis with resultant "slouching" posture. It could also cause compression on the posterior thighs and associated blood vessels, and should be avoided. Saddle-style and tilted seats help avoid pressure to the posterior thighs, and maintained the lumbar curve of the lower back by placing the pelvis in a more neutral position, which naturally balances the spinal curves. The selection of the dental stool depended on many characteristics included seat angle, depth and style, back support, height and tilt, shoulder support, adjustability of seat height, seat fabric, stability, five casters and wide base (El-Eisa *et al*, 2008).

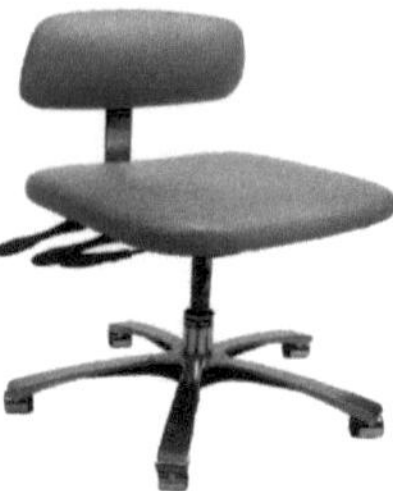

Figure10. *Traditional tilting dental stool (Royal dental). (Adopted from: Valachi 2010.Ergonomics and injury in the dental office article.pp29).*

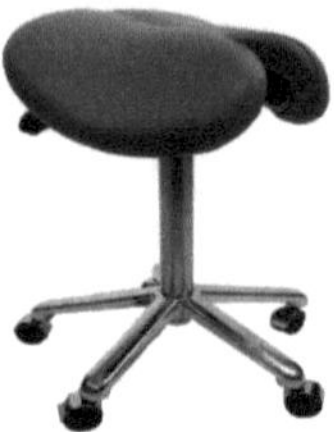

Figure 11. *Saddle- style stool (Scandex). (Adopted from: Valachi 2010. Ergonomics and injury in the dental office article.pp29).*

Back support was obtained by selecting a chair with a backrest that could be correctly adjusted for height and angulation. Lumbar support was helpful in avoiding any damaging spinal compression (as discussed above) and muscular activity, by maintaining an ergonomic spinal curve of the seated person. Tilted seats did not flatten the lower back curve as much as non-tilted stools do. The lumbar support need be only eight inches or so in height to be effective. Static supports — i.e., armrests — might offer benefits by providing support during procedures. Shoulder support was aided by armrests, which help prevent back, shoulder and neck pain. Armrests were particularly useful if the dentists were staying in one position for an extended period of time, as appeared in the figure (12) and figure (13) (El-Eisa *et al,* 2008).

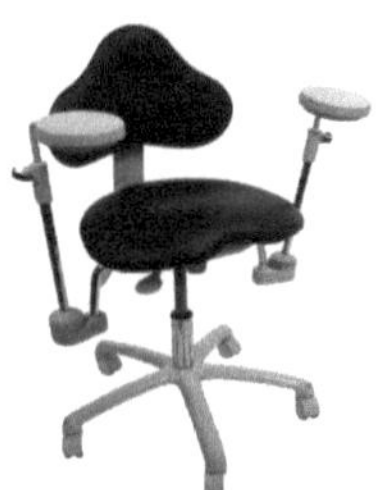

Figure 12. *Adjustable pivoting armrests and tilting seat (Ergoflex stool, Brewer) and tilted stool (Bodyguard stool, Orascoptic) . (Adopted from: Valachi 2010.Ergonomics and injury in the dental office article.pp30).*

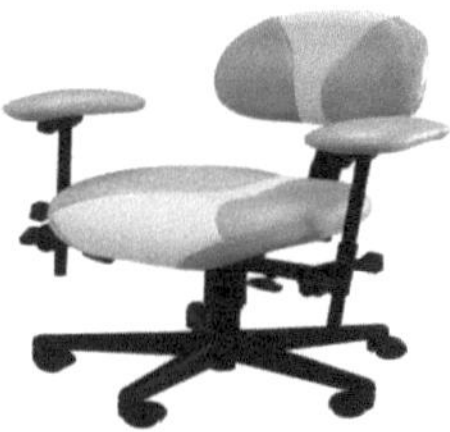

Figure13. *Armrest and titled stool (Bodyguard stool, Orascoptic). (Adopted from:Valachi 2010.Ergonomics and injury in the dental office article.pp30).*

Properly selected and adjusted, magnification devices could help prevent the dentists from gradually tilting his or her head and leaning forward over the patient as appeared in the figure (14), which could result in head and neck strain and musculoskeletal injures over time. It was important to note that inappropriate use of these aids could actually increase the risk of injury and exacerbate existing disorders. The magnification aid selected depended on a number of considerations included dentists preference, available space, magnification requirement, prior exposure to the device, learning curve and Cost. Available magnification devices included the procedure scope, Loupes (or telescopes), magnification lenses (reading glasses) and dental operating microscopes as appeared in the figure (15) (Branson, Bray, Gadbury, Holt, & Keselyak, 2008).

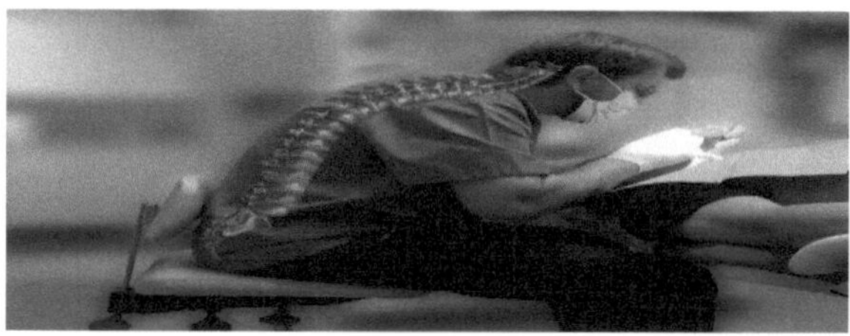

Figure14. *Flexed posture without magnification. (Adopted from: Valachi 2010.Ergonomics and injury in the dental office article.pp31).*

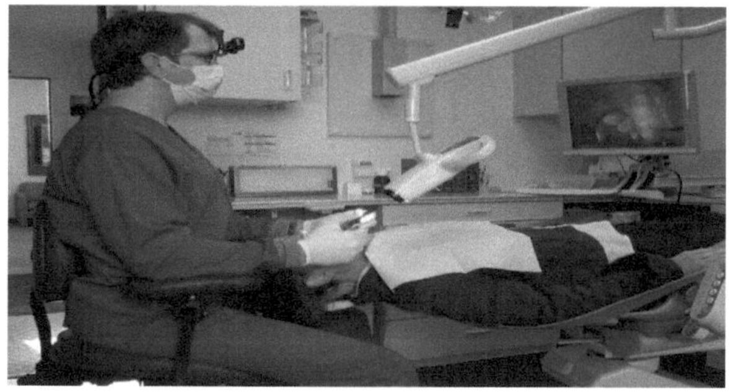

Figure 15. *Procedure scope (Magnavu); Orascoptic Bodyguard chair. (Adopted from: Valachi 2010.Ergonomics and injury in the dental office article.pp31).*

Dental Loupes (or telescopes) had been the most frequently used forms of magnification as shown in the figure (16). They offered from two to five times magnification. With appropriate selection, well-adjusted loops could enhance posture and position during procedures, resulting in improved ergonomics. Forward head posture should be no more than 25 degrees during use. Proper fitting of Loupes was essential to optimize their influence on vision and posture. It was crucial in selecting any magnification aid first to determine the optimal working posture/position and second to choose a magnification aid based on this position that had the appropriate declination angle, field of vision and working distance (Maillet *et al,* 2008).

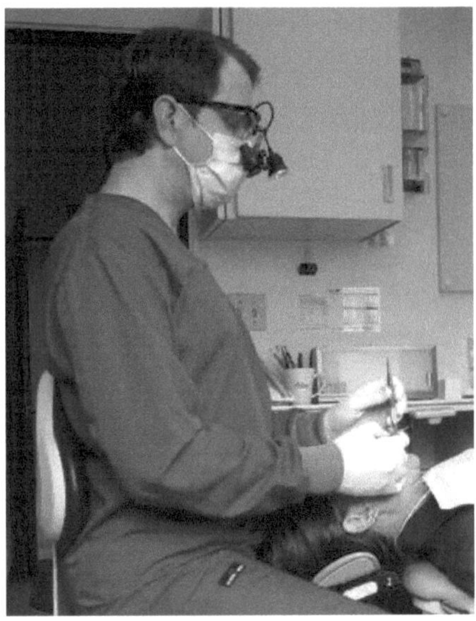

Figure 16. *Dental Loupes, appropriate chair and good posture. (Adopted from: Valachi 2010.Ergonomics and injury in the dental office article.pp33).*

Preventive health care measures for the chemical work-related health risk factors:-

Chemical health risk factors were of major concern in a dental practice. Dental nurses and dentists must be aware of the preventive health care measures that followed to eliminate the risks of the chemical hazards. Knowledge of chemicals that presented a hazard in their handling and use was essential for all staff. A list of chemicals and materials that were potentially hazardous might be identified. It should not be regarded as definitive and from time to time additions and deletions would be required. Different practices would have different lists. Each practice should maintain an up-to-date list of chemicals on the premises along with the appropriate Material Safety Data Sheets (MSDS) as appeared in the figure (17) (Smith *et al*, 2010).

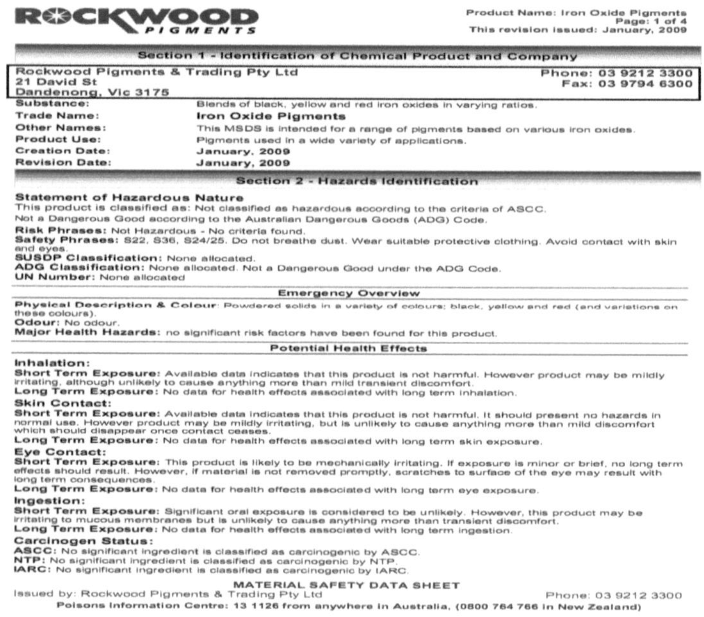

Figure 17. *Example of Material Safety Data Sheet. (Adopted from: Kilford 2009. The National code of practice for the preparation of material safety data sheet journal.pp2).*

Material Safety Data Sheets contained information on products, hazardous to health, such as storage and safe handling requirements, precautions for use, first-aid procedures, and physical properties. The manufacturers or importers were required to make an MSDS available in any place of work where a product hazardous to health was used.

The dental nurses might ensure that a current MSDS or other written information of equivalent quality, such as a product safety card, is accessible to staff working with or who were exposed to chemicals in the course of their duties. The MSDS register must be reviewed on an annual basis and documented that this has been completed (Smith *et al,* 2010).

All dental nurses and dentists would receive training in the use and safe handling of chemical disinfectants (e.g. Formaldehyde, hydrogen peroxide) before they were required to handle these disinfectants. This training would be reviewed and updated where appropriate. All such training would be recorded. All staff would be trained to emphasize the importance of disinfectants being stored in a secure manner to prevent unlawful access. Any new disinfectants coming into the practice would be advised of any possible likelihood of exposure to hazardous material or situations, and how to deal with this should it arise. List all hazardous materials used in the practice in a hazardous chemical register and update as necessary (Smith *et al,* 2010).

The dental nurses must ensure the safety storage of chemical disinfectants by ensuring that all containers had labels to show chemical identity and appropriate hazard wanting where possible, included first-aid information. Care must be taken that incompatible chemicals were not stored together. Chemical compatibility information was included on the MSDS. Hazard potential depends on the amount of exposure and individual variables. In most dental practices amounts of chemicals were small and risks were correspondingly small. All chemicals used in a dental practice must be stored in a manner that prevent accidental or unlawful access, e.g. secures/ lockable cupboard or filing cabinet (Smith *et al,* 2010).

All materials/drugs used in a dental practice must be stored in a manner that prevents accidental or unlawful access, e.g. secures/lockable cupboard or filing cabinet. In storage, take special precautions to avoid child access. Follow your staff's protocol for disposal of expired and obsolete drugs. Keys to any lockable cupboards might be kept in a safe/secure place and available to dental staff only. In addition to mercury storage and handling, the mercury poising could be minimized by careful handling, collecting the waste part of amalgam in a closed container and subjecting it to recycle, use of the proper evacuation system and avoiding the direct physical contact. Also sealed amalgam capsules use with lower mercury level, water irrigation and high suction, good ventilation and proper collection, and discarding of amalgam had substantially diminished the mercury dangers (Isfahan, 2012).

The incidence of contact dermatitis was high among the dental nurses and dentists as a result of frequent wearing of latex gloves and PPE that contained latex components. In order to reduce the risk of latex product-associated adverse reactions in both dental nurses and dentists, federal regulatory agencies such as the Food and Drug Administration (FDA), NIOSH, OSHA and CDC had been instituted policies and recommendations regarding appropriate selection of products, work practices to reduce risk, staff education, and the monitoring of allergic symptoms. For example, the FDA requires all medical/dental products and/or devices that contained latex to be clearly labeled "contains latex" (Isfahan, 2012).

In the newly released Guidelines for Infection Control in Dental Healthcare Settings, CDC, (2010b) suggested a number of protocols to decline and manage latex sensitivity and associated adverse reactions in dentistry. Accordingly, dental nurses and dentists should be familiar with the signs and symptoms of latex sensitivity. A physician should evaluate dental nurses and dentists were experiencing symptoms of latex allergy, because further exposure could result in a serious allergic reaction, procedures should be in place for minimizing latex-related health problems in dental nurses and dentists while protecting them from infectious materials. These procedures included reducing exposures to latex-containing materials, using appropriate work practices, training and educating dental nurses and dentists, monitoring symptoms, and substituting non-latex products when appropriate.

<u>Preventive health care measures for the biological work-related health risk factors:-</u>

Infection-control was important in the practice of dentistry because dental nurses and dentists were exposed to a wide variety of microorganisms via blood, oral, or respiratory secretions. These microorganisms might include the exposure to the biological health risk factors as HBV, HCV, HIV and other respiratory tract infection or disease. The mode of transmission of such exposures primarily due to injury from needles and sharp instruments. Manipulations without barrier precautions also increase the risk of infection (CDC, 2010b).

A set of infection–control strategies common to all dental care delivery settings should reduced the risk of transmission of infectious diseases, especially those caused by blood borne pathogens such as HBV, HCV, and HIV. Infected patients cannot be identified by medical history, by physical examination, or by laboratory tests. Therefore, all blood, saliva, and other patient's fluids should be considered potentially infectious. Standard precautions must be followed routinely in the care of all dental patients. The recommended infection-control practices include hand washing, wearing of personal protective equipments, protective clothing and vaccination for the dental nurses and dentists (CDC, 2010b).

Hand hygiene (e.g., hand washing, hand antisepsis, or surgical hand antisepsis) substantially reduced pathogens on the hands and is considered the single most critical measure for reducing the risk of transmission of organisms to dental nurses and dentists. The preferred method of hand hygiene depended on the type of procedure, the degree of contamination, and the desired persistence of antimicrobial action on the skin. For routine dental procedures washing hands with plain, non anti- microbial soap is sufficient. For more invasive procedures, such as cutting of gum or tissue, hand antisepsis with either an antiseptic solution or alcohol–based hand rub was recommended. If available, waterless alcohol hand rub/gel could be used in place of hand washing if hands were not visibly soiled (CDC, 2010b).

For oral surgical procedures, surgical hand antisepsis must be performed before wearing surgical gloves by either using an anti- microbial soap and water, or soap and water, followed by drying hands and application of an alcohol–based surgical hand–rub product with persistent activity, the purpose of surgical hand antisepsis was to eliminate transient flora and reduce resident flora to prevent introduction of organisms in the operative wound. Also the indications for hand hygiene included at the beginning of the working day with an antiseptic solution, if available, otherwise plain non–anti microbial soap is sufficient; before wearing gloves; between each patient; after glove removal; when hands were visibly soiled; after bare handed touching of inanimate objects likely to be contaminated by blood, saliva, or respiratory secretions; and at the end of the day (Kohn *et al,* 2010).

Dental nurses and dentists must be worn PPE such as masks, protective eyewear, face shields, protective clothing, and disposable gloves when performing procedures which caused a risk of contact with blood, blood contaminated saliva or mucous membranes as appeared in the figure (18). For protection of personnel and patients in dental–care settings, medical gloves (latex or vinyl) always must be worn by dental nurses and dentists when there was a potential for contacting blood, blood–contaminated saliva, or mucous membranes. Non sterile gloves were appropriate for examinations and other nonsurgical procedures; sterile gloves should be used for surgical procedures (Kohn *et al*, 2010).

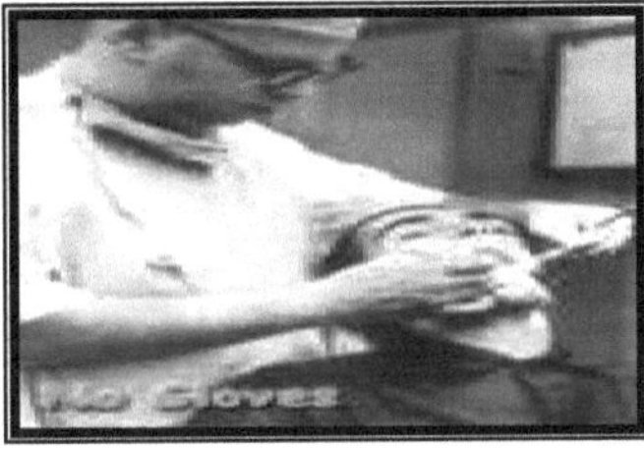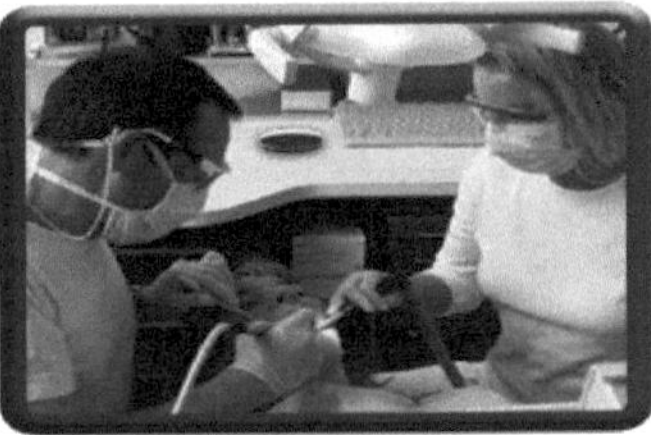

Figure18. *Comparison between dentist wearing personal protective equipment and another one not wearing it. (Adopted from: Saleh 2010. Knowledge, Attitude and Practice Toward blood borne diseases among dental health care workers thesis. pp61).*

Before treatment of each patient, dental nurses and dentists should wash their hands, and then put on new gloves; gloves must be in the correct size; after treatment of each patient or before leaving the dental operatory dental nurses and dentists should remove and discard gloves, then washed their hands. Dental nurses and dentists always should wash their hands and reglove between patients. Gloves that were torn, cut, or punctured should be removed as soon as possible and washed hands before regloving. Surgical or examination gloves should not be washed before use; nor should they be washed, disinfected, or sterilized for reuse. Washing of gloves may cause "wicking" (penetration of liquids through undetected holes in the gloves) and was not recommended (CDC, 2010b).

Protective eye wear must be worn during procedures that involved splash and spatter of saliva and blood. Eyewear protected the eyes from damage and microbes which could be transmitted through the conjunctiva. Face shields served as barriers to protect the mucous membranes of the eye, nose, and mouth from spatter. Eyewear and face shields should be washed with an appropriate cleaning agent and when visibly soiled, disinfected between patients. Masks served as barriers in dental procedures to protect the mucous membranes of the nose and mouth from spatter. Dental nurses and dentists should routinely wear face masks during dental treatment and should change them when they become wet (i.e., typically between patient treatments). Use a new mask for each patient. Masks should not be worn outside the dental operatory (CDC, 2010b).

Protective clothing such as reusable or disposable gowns, laboratory coats, or uniforms should be worn when clothing is likely to be soiled with blood or other body fluids. Clothing typically must have a high neck and long sleeves to protect the arms if splash and spatter occurred. Protective clothing should be changed at least daily and definitely when visibly soiled. Clothing must be removed before leaving the workplace reusable clothing should be washed using a normal laundry cycle. In addition to CDC recommends that all workers, including dental nurses and dentists, who might be exposed to blood or blood–contaminated substances in an occupational setting, should be vaccinated for HBV. Dental nurses and dentists also are at risk for exposure to and possible transmission of other vaccine-preventable diseases; accordingly, vaccination against influenza, measles, mumps, rubella, and tetanus may be appropriate for dental nurses and dentists (CDC, 2010b).

<u>Preventive health care measures for the psychological work-related health risk factors:-</u>

As well as, the dental nurses and dentists must be coping with the psychological health risk factors as coping with work related stress. The goal of coping with stress was to offset the negative effects of stress by using appropriate coping strategies. Coping could be done by, participating in activities that make to feel better, going to movies or participating in religious, social or other activities. Stress management workshops were focusing on stress relievers might include deep breathing exercises; progressive, effective relaxation of areas of the body; listening to audiotapes of oral instructions on how to relax; meditation; information on the topics of practice and business management, time management, communication and interpersonal skills (Babji *et al*, 2011).

These workshops should be structured to help improve dental nurses and dentists' coping skills and equip them to deal more effectively with the stressors intrinsic to the profession. Physical exercise, such as regular walking or working out at a health club, cannot be underestimated as a stress reliever. Such activities resulted in burning up the additional supply of adrenaline those resulted from stress, and they allow the body's functions to return to a more normal state. Physical exercise help develop greater self-esteem, self-control and self-discipline (Rada & Johnson, 2011).

People's personalities and temperaments have a significant impact on their perceptions of stress. Those who have strong, positive self-images and know how to relax so as to reduce mental and emotional pressures also cope better with stress, as do people who were open to being helped by others. Stressors such as failing to meet personal expectations, seeing more patients for financial reasons, working quickly to see as many patients as possible for financial reasons, earning enough money to meet the lifestyle needs and being perceived as an inflicting of pain were all stress-producing situations and had to be taken care. Break the large task into small ones. Application of relaxation, hypnosis and desensitization technique help in stress management. Anxiety disorder and depression could be treated with anti-anxiety or antidepressant drugs and psychotherapy (Regier, Row, & Narrow, 2011).

Brar & Karar, (2011) explained that in everyday clinical practice the dental nurses and dentists have to adapt an individual attitude towards a patient, depending on his/her mental state & personality. A stress situation was produced if the patient was not satisfied with the treatment rendered by the dental nurse or the dentist. In most cases, the knowledge of psychology, good communication skills and the establishment of a proper relation between dental nurses or dentist and the patient were the most crucial factors which decide the outcome of the treatment. Good communication between the dental nurse or dentist and the patient had a positive influence upon a stricter observance of the dentist's recommendations with the patient. The course of the dental nurse or dentist patient relations significantly reflected the patient's health action and result of treatment.

Puriene, (2011) found that emotional support might be gained from co-workers that were why the numbers of burnout syndrome might decrease in the larger practice groups. Conversely, a particular characteristic of private practice was the high level of control. It allowed the dental nurses and dentists to have control over their working conditions, a factor which was reported to help reduce stress levels. It was also related to income, autonomy and the match between technical aspirations and practical outcomes. Strong coping patterns result when dental nurses and dentists maintain a balance of time and responsibility, satisfaction in work and family activity, regular communication, sharing of decision making, good physical health, and the inclusion of an active exercise program within multiple demands on their time.

Furthermore, superiors in a hierarchy are available for support and help when necessary, which could substantially alleviate anxiety. This argument was counterbalanced by the issues of autonomy and control. Large organizations were able to deal with issues such as staff discipline, communication with other organizations and financial control. In small organizations such as general dental practice, the stress associated with these

46

activities was concentrated to a small number of people, frequently the dental nurses and dentists. Differences of individual responses to stress and stress management might be attributable to personality factors and differences in coping styles, and tend to support the hypothesis that stress was a unique, perceptual and experimental phenomenon (Brand & Chalmar, 2011).

Relying on the previous literatures the dental nurses and dentists were constantly exposed to various work related health risk factors include physical, mechanical, chemical, biological and psychological specific to the profession, it could develop and intensify with years. In many cases they result in diseases and disease complexes, some of which were regarded as work related illnesses. Awareness regarding theses work related health risk factors and implementation of preventive health care measures to various work related health risk factors include physical, mechanical, chemical, biological and psychological could provide a safe work environment for all dental nurses and dentists. There was also a need for continuous education programs about the work health risk factors and the preventive health care measures; it's considered one of the roles of the occupational health nurse so that the dental nurses and dentists could update themselves with the latest and newer techniques and materials (Gamphir, Singh, Sharma, Brar, & Karar, 2011).

<u>The role of occupational health nurse:-</u>

According to WHO, (2011d) prevention of health risk factors in the workplace was central to the practice of occupational health nurse as a profession. The occupational health nurses played an important role in maintaining the health and safety of health care worker through the three levels of prevention. Primary level of prevention includes both health promotion and work- related injury or disease prevention. The health promotion described as the following, it was the science and art of helping workers changed their lifestyle to move toward a state of optimal health, which in turn was defined as a balance of physical, emotional, social, spiritual and intellectual health. Lifestyle change could be facilitated through a combination of efforts to enhance awareness, change behaviors and create environments that support good health practices. Of the three, supportive environments would probably have the greatest impact in producing lasting changes.

The work- related injury or disease prevention began with recognition of health risk factor, a disease, injury or an environmental hazard and was followed by measures to protect as many staff as possible from the harmful consequences of that risk. The occupational health nurse used a variety of primary prevention methods, with one-on-one interaction as an important strategy for evaluating risk reduction behavior for staff. The occupational health nurse had daily contact with numerous staff for many reasons (e.g., assessment and treatment of episodic illness or injury and health surveillance); therefore this was an important method for promoting health (Neis & Ewen, 2011).

However, similar to community health nursing professional, occupational health nurses plan, develop, implement, and evaluate aggregate- focused intervention strategies. The occupational health nurse planned and implemented programs such as weight and cholesterol reduction, ergonomics training, and smoking cessation. Performing "walk-through" in the workplace on a regular basis, recognizing potential and existing health risk factors, and maintaining communications with safety and industrial hygiene resources would continue to be critical work of the occupational health nurse (Shortdge & McCauly, 2011).

Types of non-occupational programs included in the dental practice area of primary prevention are cancer awareness, personal safety, immunization, disease or injury prevention, retirement health, stress management, and relaxation techniques. Occupational health programs could include topics such as emergency response, first aid and infection control programs, right to know training, immunization programs, programs for the application of preventive health care measures, ergonomics, and other programs targeted to specific health risk factors identified in the workplace (Neis & Ewen, 2011).

Secondary prevention strategies were aimed at early diagnosis, early treatment interventions, and attempts to limit disability. The focus at this level of prevention was an identification of health needs, health problems and staff at risk. As with primary prevention, the occupational health nurse used a number of different secondary prevention strategies, also added that by providing direct care for episodic illness and injury, the occupational health nurse was afforded the opportunity to conduct assessments and provided treatment and referrals for a variety of physical and psychological conditions (Shortdge & McCauly, 2011).

The occupational health nurse could offer health screenings for dental nurses and dentists, which were designed for early detection of disease, at the work site with relative ease and at minimal cost. Screenings might focus on hearing impairment, cancer, eye injury, and contact dermatitis, any infectious diseases (e.g. Hepatitis B, Hepatitis C, and respiratory infection). Secondary prevention efforts provided by the occupational health nurse include pre-placement, periodic, and job transfer evaluations to ensure that the dental nurse or the dentist was being placed or was continuing to work in a job that is safe for that dental nurse or the dentist. The pre-placement evaluation was performed before the dental nurse or the dentist began employment in a new dental health care setting or was placed in different dental setting. The evaluation was a baseline examination that consisted of a medical history, an occupational health history, and a physical assessment that should be targeted the type of work that the dental nurse or the dentist would perform (WHO, 2011d).

The examination might also include medical tests to determine specific organ functions that might be affected by exposure to existing agents in the dental nurse or dentist workplace. For example, if the dental nurse or dentist was working with a chemical substance (e.g. Amalgam) that was a known contain mercury and could be led to mercury toxicity, baseline blood and urine mercury tests may be appropriate to determine the current health status of the dental nurse and dentist and their ability to handle this specific chemical exposure (Nies & Ewen, 2011).

Nies & Ewen, (2011) also clarified that Periodic assessments usually occur at a regular interval (e.g., annual and biannual) and were based on specific protocols for the dental nurse and dentist who were exposed to substances or irritants such as mercury, anesthetic gases, noise, or various chemical disinfectants. Also for the dental nurse and dentist who were exposed to needle stick or sharp instrument injuries, who frequently used of latex and who frequently stand or sitting for a long period of time. In addition to examinations of the dental nurse and dentist transferring to other clinical settings was critical to document any changes in health that might have occurred while he/ she was working in a specific area or with specific process. Activities must continue to focus on prevention and early detection by increasing awareness of the incidence of other health conditions such as hepatitis B.

On the tertiary prevention, the occupational health nurse played a key role in the rehabilitation and restoration of the dental nurse and dentist to an optimal level of functioning. Strategies included case management, negotiation of workplace accommodations, and counseling and support for dental nurse and dentist who would continue to be affected by chronic disease (e.g. Hepatitis C). Also, she completed a risk assessment, devise the rehabilitation program, monitor progress and communicate with the dental nurses and dentists, coordinated health care services for the dental nurses and dentists from the onset of injury or illness to a safe return to work or an optimal alternative (WHO, 2011d).

The occupational health nurse might fulfill several, often interrelated and complementary roles in workplace health management as described by WHO, (2011d) including: Clinician, Specialist, Manager, Coordinator, Adviser, Health educator, Counselor and Researcher. According to the primary level of prevention, the occupational health nurse acted as a clinician: Primary prevention the occupational health nurse was skilled in primary prevention of injury or disease. The nurse might identify the need for, assess and plan interventions to, for example, modify working environments, systems of work or change working practices in order to reduce the risk of hazardous exposure.

Occupational health nurses were skilled in considering factors, such as human behavior and habits in relation to actual working practices. The nurse could also collaborate in the identification, conception and correction of work factors, the choice of individual protective equipment, prevention of industrial injuries and diseases, as well as providing advice in matters concerning protection of the environment. Because of the occupational health nurses close association with the workers, and knowledge and experience in the working environment, they were in a good position to identify early changes in working practices, identify workers' concerns over health and safety, and by presenting these to management in an independent objective manner can be the catalyst for changes in the workplace that led to primary prevention (WHO, 2011d).

Occupational health nurses were skilled in assessing client's health care needs, established a nursing diagnosis and formulated appropriate nursing care plans, in conjunction with the patient or client groups, to meet those needs. Nurses could then implement and evaluate nursing interventions designed to achieve the core objectives. The nurse had a prominent role in assessing the needs of individuals and groups, and had the ability to analyze, interpret, plan and implement strategies to achieve specific goals. By using the nursing process the nurse contributes to workplace health management and by so doing help to improve the health of the working population at the enterprise level. Nursing diagnosis was a holistic concept that did not focu solely on the treatment of a specific disease, but rather considers the whole person and their health care needs in the broadest context. It was a health based model rather than a disease based model and nurses had the skills to apply this approach to the working populations they serve (WHO, 2011d).

Also, her role as a clinician to give advice on a wide range of health issues, and particularly on their relationship to working ability, health and safety at work or where modifications to the job or working environment could be made to take account of the changing health status of employees. In many respects employers were not solely concerned with only those conditions that were directly caused by work, but do want their occupational health staff to help address any health related problems that might arise that might influence the employees attendance or performance at work, and many employees appreciate this level of help being provided to them at the workplace because it was so convenient for them. In particular the development of health care services to men at work, younger populations and those from ethnic groups can be most effective in reaching these sometimes difficult to reach populations (WHO, 2011d).

The specialist occupational health nurse might be involved, with senior management in the enterprise, in developing the workplace health policy and strategy, included aspects of occupational health, workplace health promotion and environmental health management. The occupational health nurse was a good position to advise management on the implementation, monitoring and evaluation of workplace health management strategies and to participate fully in each of these stages. The possibility to perform that role would depend upon the level of nursing education, skills and experience (Klein, Freeman, Taylor, & Stevens, 2005).

Also, occupational health nurses could play an essential role in health assessment for fitness to work, pre-employment or pre-placement examinations, periodic health examinations and individual health assessments of lifestyle risk factors. Collaboration with an occupational physician might be necessary in many instances, depending upon exiting legislation and accepted practice. The nurse could also play an important role in the workplace where informal requests for information, advice on health care matters and health related problems come to light. The nurse was able to observe the individual or group of workers in relation to exposure to a particular hazard and initiate appropriate targeted health assessment where necessary. These activities were often, but not exclusively, undertaken in conjunction with the medical adviser so that where problems were identified a safe system for onward referral exists (Klein *et al*, 2005).

The occupational health nurse often had close contact with the workers and was aware of changes to the working environment. Because of the nurses' expertise in health and in the effects of work on health they were in a good position to be involved in hazard identification. Hazards might arise due to new processes or working practices or might arise out of informal changes to existing processes and working practices that the nurse could readily identify and assessed the likely risk from. This activity required and presupposed regular and frequent workplace visits by the occupational health nurse to maintain an up to date knowledge and awareness of working processes and practices (Klein *et al*, 2005).

In some cases the occupational health nurse might act as the manager of the multidisciplinary occupational health team, directing and coordinating the work of other occupational health professionals. The occupational health nurse manager might have management responsibility for the whole of the occupational health team, or the nursing staff or management responsibility for specific program. The nurse manager might be the budget holder for the department and would have the skills necessary to sit alongside other line managers within the organization and contribute to organizational development. Also, the occupational health nurse could have a role in administration. Maintaining medical and nursing records, monitoring expenditure, staffing levels and skill mix within the department, and might have responsibility for managing staff involved in administration (WHO, 2011d).

The occupational health nurse was acting as a coordinator, could draw together all of the professionals involved in the occupational health team. In many instances the nurse would be the only member of the team who was permanently employed by the enterprise or present on a particular site. Therefore, they had a unique position and had access to valuable information that could be used to help shape and direct the occupational health program. In this role the nurse would exercise skills in communication, planning, involvement, management and in organizing the professional team (Klein *et al*, 2005).

The occupational health nurse had a role in worker education. This might be within existing training programs or those programs that were developed specifically by occupational health nurses to, for example, inform, educate and train workers in how to protect themselves from occupational hazards, non-occupational but workplace preventable diseases or to raise awareness of the importance of good environmental health management practices (Klein *et al*, 2005).

Health education as one of the key prerequisites of workplace health promotion was an integral aspect of the occupational health nurses' role. In some countries the nurse was required to support activities aimed at adoption of healthier lifestyles within an on-going health promotion process, as well as participate in health and safety activities. Occupational health nurses could carry out a needs assessment for health promotion within the enterprise, prioritize activities in consultation with management and workers, develop and plan appropriate interventions, deliver or coordinate the delivery of health promotion strategies and could play a valuable role in evaluating the delivery and achievements of the health promotion strategy (Klein *et al*, 2005).

Occupational health nurses involved in workplace health management could sometimes be asked to act as advisers to management and staff on the development of workplace health policies and practices, and could fulfill an advisory role by participating in, for example, health and safety committee meetings, health promotion meetings, and might be called upon to provide independent advice to managers or workers who had specific concerns over health related risks. Also, Occupational health nurses act in an advisory role when seeing individuals who might have problems that, whilst not directly related to work may affect future work attendance or performance. The nurse might be involved in advising individuals to seek advice from their own family doctor or general practitioner, or other external agency that might be better placed to assist the individual (WHO,2011d).

In the small or medium sized enterprise the occupational health nurse might be the only health care professional present most of the time and they could assist people working there in dealing with mental health and work-related stress. For many people the occupational health nurse, working at the enterprise level, might be the first point of contact with health care providers and these nurses could do much to ensure that individuals were referred to the appropriate agency. Where the nurse had been trained in using counseling or reflective listening skills they might utilize these skills in delivering care to individuals or groups. As part of this approach, there should be opportunities for the nurse to receive ongoing supervision and support and to have access to additional professional services to which particularly difficult cases could be referred or where additional expertise was needed in order to help the individual or group (Ethridge, MacKellar, & Branson, 2005).

Due to the close working relationship which occupational health nurses had with the working population, and because of the nurses' position of trust, occupational health nurses were often approached for advice on personal problems. The nurse could use listening techniques and problem solving skills developed through nurse education and training to meet this need. The nurse could act as a useful resource for the organization and where necessary, refer individuals on to the appropriate, skilled agencies to help them with their personal problems. This might be a clinical specialist such as physicians or psychologists, or two counselors, employee assistance programs, etc. (Ethridge *et al*, 2005).

A specialist occupational health nurse would need to be well skilled in undertaking a nurse based health needs assessment at both the individual and the organizational level. This type of assessment could be used as the basis for individual case management or occupational health program planning. Occupational health nurses might use research based skills in carrying out the assessment, in handling the data generated in the assessment and in interpreting the results and advising management acting as a member of the multidisciplinary team. Nurses were becoming increasingly familiar with both quantitative and qualitative research methodologies, and could apply these in occupational health nursing practice. In the main, occupational health nurses working at the enterprise level, were more likely to use simple survey techniques, or semi-structured interviews, and to use descriptive statistical techniques in their presentation of the data (Ethridge *et al,* 2005).

Increasingly, all health care providers were using an evidence-based approach to practice that required the professional to seek the best available information on which to base their practice. Occupational health nurses were skilled in searching the literature, reviewing the evidence available, which might be in the form of practice guidelines or protocols, and were applying these guidance documents in a practical situation. Occupational health nurses should be well skilled in presenting the evidence, were identifying gaps in current knowledge, and allowing others to review critically the implementation of care plans based on their assessment of the evidence (Ethridge *et al,* 2005).

As was concluded from the role of occupational health nurse that the complex, highly dynamic processes used by occupational health nurses to deliver health care interventions to working populations in diverse organizations cannot be described simply in a list of core competencies, but those described here represented some of the core competencies and areas of knowledge that occupational health nurses already use in some countries. An individual nurse, or group of nurses, might not be skilled in all of these areas of practice equal, but would develop and mold their practice to meet the needs of the populations they serve. In different countries, different health care systems were in operation and occupational health nurses practicing in those settings would tailor their efforts to complement the existing health care systems (WHO, 2011d).

CHAPTER III

Subjects and Methods

<u>Aim of the Study</u>

The aim of the study will be two folds:-

- Assess the work-related health risk factors among dental nurses and dentists.

- Assess the preventive health care measures applied among dental nurses and dentists.

<u>Research Questions</u>

To fulfill aim of this study, the following research questions were formulated:

1.   What are the work-related health risk-factors that prevailing among dental nurses and dentists?

2.   What are preventive health care measures that are applied by dental nurses and dentists?

<u>Research design</u>

A descriptive cross-sectional research design was utilized in this study; such design fits the nature of the problem under investigation.

<u>Sample</u>

A convenient sample of dental nurses and dentists at faculty of oral and dental medicine at Cairo University constituted the subjects of the study. The total sample reached 50 dental nurses and out of 200 of deputy, demonstrator and assistant lecturer dentists who were asked to participate in the study 150 dentists accepted to participate. (At the old dental educational building, two dental nurses and twenty dentists were chosen from the diagnosis clinic another two dental nurses and six dentists were chosen from the extraction clinic, eight dental nurses and thirty dentists from the five treatment clinics. At the pediatric dental educational building, two dental nurses and eleven dentists were chosen from the diagnosis clinic another nine dental nurses and forty dentists were chosen from the four treatment clinics and two dental nurses, six dentists from the treatment clinic for mental retarded children and no one of dental nurses or dentists were chosen from general anesthesia unit. At the new dental educational building, four dental nurses and four dentists from the two orthodontic clinic another four dental nurses and four dentists from the fixed prosthodontic clinic, three dental nurses and four dentists were chosen from the operative clinic and fourteen dental nurses and twenty-five dentists from the eleven out-patient clinics for treatment for free and paid).

Exclusion Criteria:

- Pregnant women.

- Dental nurses and dentists who complained from chronic diseases.

- Dental nurses and dentists who exceed 40 years.

<u>Setting</u>

The study was conducted at the dental clinics of the faculty of oral and dental medicine at the Elkasr Eleiny educational hospital. The faculty consisted of three buildings as shown in (figure 19); the first building was an old dental educational building and included eleven dental clinics for diagnosis, extraction, and treatment. The second building was a pediatric dental clinic and included five dental clinics for diagnosis and treatment for free or paid and unit for general anesthesia. The third building was new dental educational building that included five clinics for orthodontics, fixed prosthondontics and operative clinic for free or paid.

Three tools were used for data collection that designed after extensive review of literature by the investigator.

<u>First tool</u>: Sociodemographic questionnaire:-

Structured questionnaire was developed by investigator and cover the following items:

- Demographic characteristics of dental nurses and dentists as: age, gender, marital status, level of education and years of experience in dental clinics.

<u>Second tool</u>: work-related health risk factors questionnaire: theses questionnaire was developed by investigator to cover dental nurses and dentists about the following items:

a) Workplace health risk factors prevailed among dental nurses and dentists as latex allergy, eye injury, low back pain, Hepatitis B and emotional exhaustion.

b) Dental nurses and dentists' knowledge about five types of work related health risk factors and its causes as: Biological work related health risk factors as Hepatitis B&C, Chemical work related health risk factors as latex allergy, Physical work related health risk factors as eye injury and percutaneous exposure incidents, Mechanical work related health risk factors as low back pain and neck pain, Psychological work related health risk factors as emotional exhaustion and depersonalization.

The score of knowledge was one (1) for a correct answer and zero for an incorrect answer or unknown answer. The total score of knowledge reached 32 scores. Then calculated level of knowledge classified into three levels as: good, when score 90% or more of the total score. Satisfactory, when score 75% to less than 90% of the total score. Unsatisfactory, when score was less than 75% of the total score.

<u>Third tool</u>: Structured observational checklist developed by the investigator and used to assess the preventive health care measures applied by dental nurses and dentists in dental clinics regarding work-related health risk factors as biological, chemical, physical, mechanical and psychological preventive health care measures.

The scores of observable checklist for dental nurses and dentists were one (1) for done practice and zero for not done practice. The total scores for dental nurses' practice were 44 while 50 for dentists, these differences in the total scores aroused from exclusion of not applicable items either for nurses or dentists. The calculated observed practice was classified into three levels as: Good, when scores 90% or more of the total score. Satisfactory, when scores were 75% to less than 90% of the total score. Unsatisfactory, as when score was less than 75% of the total score.

Content Validity

The content validity was done for each item of developed tools by four experts in the field of community health nursing department, Faculty of Nursing, Cairo University and one expert in dental public health, Faculty of Oral and Dental medicine, Cairo University. Then the recommended modification was done by the investigator.

Pilot study

A pilot study was conducted on 10% of the sample size to assess the applicability and the clarity of the tools to estimate the time needed for completion of tools and questions need to add or omit. The necessary modifications were done with the tools based on the pilot study. Dental nurses and dentists participated in the pilot study were excluded from the study sample.

Ethical and legal considerations

A written ethical approval was obtained from the ethical committee of scientific research at the Faculty of Nursing, Cairo University. In addition, an official permission to conduct the proposed study was obtained from; Vice Dean of the postgraduates and research studies at Faculty of Nursing and an official permission was obtained from the college council of the Faculty of Oral and Dental Medicine. A written formal consent was obtained from the dental nurses and dentists after explaining to them, the aim of the study, its benefits and risks, duration of study and data collection tools. The investigator informed the dental nurses and dentists that all gathered data considered confidential. The investigator also informed them about their rights to withdraw from the study at any time without giving any reason and without any pressure from the head of department.

Procedure

Based on a review of literature, the tools were developed and approval was obtained from the ethical committee of the Faculty of Nursing Cairo University, initial approval was obtained on March 2014.

Permission was obtained from the vice dean of postgraduate and research studies of the Faculty of Oral and Dental medicine Cairo University. Then an official permission to conduct the proposed study was obtained from the college council of both Faculties of Nursing and Faculty of Oral and Dental medicine Cairo University. Dental nurses and dentists were invited to participate in the study, and the investigator explained the aims of the study to each dental nurse and dentist to gain their cooperation then written consent was obtained.

62

The structured questionnaire was completed by dental nurses and dentists in the presence of the investigator in the dental clinic. Practices of dental nurses and dentists were observed by the investigator regarding the application of preventive health care measures. Nearly 7 to 8 of dental nurses and 20 to 25 dentists were participated and observed during their work in the clinic per month from 9 am till 2 pm. The time spent to fill the questionnaire by each dental nurse or dentist ranged between 10 to 15 minutes. The time spent to fill the observational checklist after two times of visiting the clinic were 240 hours. The study was conducted from June till November 2014. After collection of the data, the written informed consents were submitted for the second time to the ethical committee for evaluation and final approval was obtained on December 2014.

Statistical Analysis

On completion of data collection, data were tabulated and analyzed using statistical package for social sciences (SPSS) program version 20 relevant statistical analysis was done to test the obtained data. Descriptive and inferential statistics were performed such as mean and standard deviation; frequency; percentage and correlation coefficient. Probability (p-value) less than 0.05 was considered significant and less than 0.001 was considered as highly significant.

CHAPTER IV

Results

<u>Aim of the study:-</u>

The present study aimed at assessing the work-related health risk factors among dental nurses and dentists and to assess the preventive health care measures applied among dental nurses and dentists.

<u>Research questions:</u>

Q1:   What are the work-related health-risk factors that prevailing among dental nurses and dentists?

Q2:   What are preventive health care measures that are applied by dental nurses and dentists?

<u>The study results will be presented according to the following sequence:</u>

 Part I- Socio-demographic and work services rendered for dental nurses and dentists. (Tables 2-5)

 Part II- Work-related health risk factors that prevailing among dental nurses and dentists. (Tables 6-17 & Figures 20-21)

Part III- Preventive health care measures applied by dental nurses and dentists. (Tables 18-27& Figures 22-25)

Part IV: The relations between work-related health risk factors and preventive healthcare measures among dental nurses and dentists. (Tables 28-35)

Part I: Socio-demographic and work services rendered for dental nurses and dentists.

The socio-demographic characteristics of the dental nurses are presented in table (2), 98% are females with a mean age of 31± 5.28 years while 90% of dental nurses have secondary school nursing education and 62% of them are married. The table also reveals that, 60% of dental nurses have less than six years of work experience with the mean of 2.4 ±0.95 years.

<u>Table 2</u>

<u>*Distribution of dental nurses according to their Socio-demographic characteristics (n=50)*</u>

Socio-demographic characteristics	No.	%
Gender		
Male	1	2.0
Female	49	98.0
Age (in years)		
20-	7	14.0
25-	11	22.0
30-	14	28.0
35-40	18	36.0
Mean ± SD	31±5.28	
Marital status		
Single	18	36.0
Married	31	62.0
Widow	1	2.0
Educational level		
Secondary	45	90.0
Technical Institute	5	10.0
Bachelor	0	0.0
Years of work experience		
<1 year	7	14.0
1-5 year	23	46.0
6-10 year	11	22.0
>10 years	9	18.0
Mean ± SD	2.4±0.95	

The socio-demographic characteristics of dentists are presented in table (3), 68.8% are females with a mean age of 28.18 ± 2.51 years while 56% of dentists have master degree and 54% of them are married. The table also shows that, 62% of dentists have less than six years experience with a mean of 2.3 ±0.76 years.

Table 3

Distribution of dentists according to their Socio-demographic characteristics (n=150)

Sociodemographic characteristics	No.	%
Gender		
Male	47	31.3
Female	103	68.6
Age (in years)		
25-	104	69.3
30-34	46	30.6
Mean ± SD	28.18±2.51	
Marital status		
Single	69	46.0
Married	81	54.0
Educational level		
Bachelor	61	40.7
Master	84	56.0
Doctorate	5	3.3
Years of work experience		
< 1 year	17	11.3
1-5 years	76	50.6
6-10 years	47	31.3
>10 years	10	6.6
Mean ± SD	2.3±0.76	

Table (4) shows that, 50% of dental nurses didn't have any medical check-up while 30% of them have a medical check-up from less than 6 months. Concerning training of dental nurses, 72% of dental nurses get training from continuing education units inside the faculty while 48% of them get pre-employment training. In relation to safety of the work environment, 82% of dental nurses get vaccinated in their workplace while 50% of dental nurses express that there is safety measures in their work environment.

Table 4

Distribution of work services rendered for dental nurses (n=50)

Services rendered	No.	%
Medical check-up		
No	25	50.0
Yes:		
< 6 months	15	30.0
6-12 months	5	10.0
1 year	5	10.0
***Workplace Training**		
No	10	20.0
Yes:		
Pre-employment	24	48.0
Continuous	36	72.0
New equipment and techniques	25	50.0
***Safety of work environment**		
No	10	20.0
Yes:		
Availability of vaccination	41	82.0
Availability of safety measures	25	50.0

*Responses aren't mutually exclusive.

Table (5) indicates that, 41.3% of dentists have a medical check-up and 33.3% of
them have a medical check-up from less than 6 months. Concerning training of dentists,
33.3% of dentists get training when the faculty introduces new equipment or technique into
the clinics while 24% of them get pre-employment training. In relation to safety of the
work environment, 91% of dentists get vaccinated in their workplace while only 5.3% of
dentists express that there is safety measures in their work environment.

Table 5

Distribution of work services rendered for dentists (n=150)

Services rendered	No.	%
Medical check-up		
No	88	58.6
Yes:	65	41.3
< 6 months	50	33.3
6-12 months	10	6.6
1 year	2	1.3
***Workplace Training**		
No	50	33.3
Yes:		
Pre-employment	36	24.0
Continuous	45	30.0
New equipment and techniques	50	33.3
Safety of work environment		
No	5	3.3
Yes:		
Availability of vaccination	137	91.0
Availability of safety measures	8	5.3

*Responses aren't mutually exclusive.

Part II: Work-related health risk factors that are prevailing among dental nurses and dentists.

Table (6) reveals that, no one of dental nurses complains of biological health risk factors while 62% of dental nurses complain of latex allergy and no one of them complain of mercury toxicity. Regarding physical health risk factors, the table shows that, 40% of dental nurses complain of eye injury and 34% of them complain of PEI while only 12% of dental nurses complain of hearing difficulties. Also table (6) clarifies that, 76% of dental nurses complain of low back pain, 50% of them complain of neck pain and 40% of them complain of shoulder pain while 82% of dental nurses complain of emotional exhaustion and 28% of them complain of depersonalization and depression.

Distribution of workplace health risk factors among dental nurses (n=50)

Workplace health risk factors	No.	%
Biological health risk factors		
Hepatitis "B"	0	0.0
Hepatitis "C"	0	0.0
Chemical health risk factors		
Latex allergy	31	62.0
Mercury toxicity	0	0.0
Physical health risk factors		
Eye Injury	20	40.0
PEI	14	34.0
Hearing difficulties	6	12.0
***Mechanical health risk factors**		
Low back pain	38	76.0
Neck pain	25	50.0
Wrist pain	15	30.0
Shoulder pain	20	40.0
***Psychological health risk factors**		
Emotional Exhaustion	41	82.0
Depersonalization	14	28.0
Depression	14	28.0

*Responses are not mutually exclusive.

Table (7) reveals that, no one of the dentists complains of biological health risk factors while 53% of dentists complain of latex allergy and no one of them complain of mercury toxicity. Regarding to physical health risk factors, the table shows that 68.7% of dentists complain of eye injury and 100% of them complain of PEI while only 18.7% of dentists complain of hearing difficulties. Also table (7) shows that 93.3% of dentists complain of low back pain, 86.7% of them complain of neck pain and 82% of them complain of shoulder pain while 100% of dentists complain of emotional exhaustion while 33.3% of them complain of depersonalization and 54% of them complain of depression.

Table 7

Distribution of workplace health risk factors among dentists (n=150)

Workplace health risk factors	No.	%
Biological health risk factors		
Hepatitis "B"	0	0.0
Hepatitis "C"	0	0.0
Chemical health risk factors		
Latex Allergy	80	53.0
Mercury toxicity	0	0.0
***Physical health risk factors**		
Eye Injury	103	68.7
PEI	150	100
Hearing difficulties	28	18.7
***Mechanical health risk factors**		
Low back pain	140	93.3
Neck pain	130	86.7
Wrist pain	104	69.3
Shoulder pain	123	82.0
***Psychological health risk factors**		
Depersonalization	50	33.3
Emotional Exhaustion	150	100
Depression	81	54.0

*Responses are not mutually exclusive.

Table (8) shows that 30% of dental nurses' choose Hepatitis B as common health risk factor that affect them and 34% of dental nurses choose HIV while only 16% choose respiratory tract infection and 20% choose Hepatitis C as a common health risk factor that affect them. Regarding to the causes of biological work-related health risk factors, the table reveals that, 36% of dental nurses choose cuts by contaminated dental equipment while 44% of them choose direct contact with blood and body fluids and 20% choose inhalation of respiratory discharge.

Table 8

Dental nurses' knowledge about the biological work- related health risk factors (n=50)

Knowledge about biological risk factors	No.	%
Health risk factors		
Hepatitis B	15	30.0
Hepatitis C	10	20.0
HIV	17	34.0
Respiratory tract infection	8	16.0
Causes of health risk factors		
Cuts by contaminated dental equipment	18	36.0
Direct contact with blood and body fluids	22	44.0
Inhalation of respiratory discharge	10	20.0

Table (9) reveals that, 96.7% of dentists' choose Hepatitis B and respiratory tract infection as health risk factors that affect them while 88.7% of dentists choose HIV and 93.3% of dentists choose Hepatitis C as the most common health risk factors that affect them. Regarding the causes of biological work-related health risk factors, 100% of dentists choose needle stick injury and direct contact with blood and body fluids also 96.7% of dentists choose the inhalation of respiratory discharge.

Table 9

Dentists' knowledge about the biological work-related health risk factors (n=150)

Knowledge about biological risk factors	No.	%
***Health risk factors**		
Hepatitis B	145	96.7
Hepatitis C	140	93.3
HIV	133	88.7
Respiratory tract infection	145	96.7
***Causes of health risk factors**		
Cuts by contaminated dental equipment	150	100
Direct contact with blood and body fluids	150	100
Inhalation of respiratory discharge	145	96.7

*Responses are not mutually exclusive.

Table (10) presents dental nurses' knowledge about chemical work-related health risk factors, where 60% of dental nurses choose latex allergy as the most health risk factor that affect them and 46% of dental nurses choose mercury toxicity. Regarding the causes of chemical work-related health risk factors, the table reveals that, only 20% of dental nurses choose mercury vapors and inappropriate storage of mercury while 60% of dental nurses choose that not to wear non latex gloves as the major cause of chemical health risk factors.

Table 10

Dental nurses' knowledge about the chemical work-related health risk factors (n=50)

Knowledge about chemical risk factors	No.	%
***Health risk factors**		
Latex allergy	30	60.0
Mercury toxicity	23	46.0
Causes of health risk factors		
Mercury vapors	10	20.0
Inappropriate storage of mercury	10	20.0
Not wearing of non latex gloves	30	60.0

*Responses are not mutually exclusive.

Table (11) reveals that, 100% of dentists choose latex allergy as the most chemical health risk factors that affect them and 73.3% of dentists choose mercury toxicity. Related to causes of chemical work-related health risk factors, 47.3% of dentists choose mercury vapors and 44 % of dentists choose the inappropriate storage of mercury while 80% of dentists choose not to wear of non latex gloves is the major cause of chemical health risk factors.

Table 11

Dentists' knowledge about the chemical work-related health risk factors (n=150)

Knowledge about chemical risk factors	No.	%
***Health risk factors**		
Latex allergy	150	100
Mercury toxicity	110	73.3
***Causes of health risk factors**		
Mercury vapors	71	47.3
Inappropriate storage of mercury	66	44.0
Not wearing of non latex gloves	120	80.0

*Responses are not mutually exclusive.

It is observed from the table (12) that, 60% of dental nurses choose percutaneous exposure incident as the most physical health risk factors that affect them while only 20% choose eye injury, also 22% of dental nurses choose hearing difficulties. In relation to the causes of physical work-related health risk factors, 34% and 26% of dental nurses choose not to use sharp containers and not to use a needle stick protector respectively as the most cause of physical work-related health risk factors while only 20% of dental nurses choose that not to wear earplugs or aprons.

<u>Table 12</u>

Dental nurses' knowledge about the physical work-related health risk factors (n=50)

Knowledge about physical risk factors	No.	%
***Health risk factors**		
Eye injury	10	20.0
Percutaneous exposure incident	30	60.0
Hearing difficulties	11	22.0
Causes of health risk factors		
Not wearing of apron	10	20.0
Not wearing of earplugs	10	20.0
Not using of sharp containers	17	34.0
Not using of needle stick protector	13	26.0

*Responses are not mutually exclusive.

It is observed from the table (13) that, 100% of dentists choose percutaneous exposure incident as the most physical health risk factors affecting them and 70.7% of dentists choose eye injury while 58% of dentists choose hearing difficulties. Table (13) shows also that, 93.3% of dentists choose not using of sharp containers as the major cause of physical health risk factors, 73.3% and 66.6% of dentists choose not to wear an apron and earplugs respectively as most causes of physical health risk factors while only 28.7% of them choose not to use a needle stick protector as a cause of physical health risk factors.

Table 13

Dentists' knowledge about the physical work-related health risk factors (n=150)

Knowledge about physical risk factors	No.	%
***Health risk factors**		
Eye injury	106	70.7
Percutaneous exposure incident	150	100
Hearing difficulties	87	58.0
***Causes of health risk factors**		
Not wearing of apron	110	73.3
Not wearing of earplugs	100	66.6
Not using of sharp containers	140	93.3
Not using of needle stick protector	43	28.7

*Responses are not mutually exclusive.

Table (14) reveals that, 42% of dental nurses choose low back pain as the most mechanical health risk factors affect them while 20% of dental nurses choose neck pain. Also, 30% and 38% of dental nurses respectively choose wrist pain and shoulder pain as the most mechanical health risk factors affecting them. Regarding the causes of mechanical health risk factors, the table indicates that, 44% of dental nurses choose an incorrect sitting posture as the most cause of mechanical health risk factors and 36% of dental nurses choose an incorrect standing posture while only 20% of them choose the repetitive use of manual instrument.

<u>Table 14</u>

Dental nurses' knowledge about the mechanical work related health risk factors (n=50)

Knowledge about mechanical risk factors	No.	%
***Health risk factors**		
Low back pain	21	42.0
Neck pain	10	20.0
Wrist pain	15	30.0
Shoulder pain	19	38.0
Causes of health risk factors		
Incorrect sitting posture	22	44.0
Incorrect standing posture	18	36.0
Repetitive using of manual instrument e.g. scalars	10	20.0

*Responses are not mutually exclusive.

Table (15) reveals that 100% of dentists choose low back pain as the most health risk factor affecting them, 83.3% of dentists choose neck pain. Also, 78.8% and 80% choose wrist pain and shoulder pain, respectively as the most health risk factor that affects them. The table clarifies also that, 83.3% of dentists choose an incorrect sitting posture as the most common cause of mechanical work-related health risk factors and 82% of them choose the repetitive use of manual instrument while 73.3% of dentists choose an incorrect standing posture.

Table 15

Dentists' knowledge about the mechanical work-related health risk factors (n=150)

Knowledge about mechanical risk factors	No.	%
***Health risk factors**		
Low back pain	150	100
Neck pain	125	83.3
Wrist pain	118	78.8
Shoulder pain	120	80
***Causes of health risk factors**		
Incorrect sitting posture	125	83.3
Incorrect standing posture	110	73.3
Repetitive using of manual instrument	123	82

*Responses are not mutually exclusive.

Table (16) shows that, 52% of dental nurses choose depersonalization as the most psychological health risk factor affecting them and 28% of dental nurses choose emotional exhaustion while 22% of dental nurses choose depression. Regarding the causes of psychological work-related health risk factors, 50% of dental nurses choose an excessive workload and 36% of dental nurses choose anesthetization of patients while 26% and 20% of dental nurses respectively choose the pain and fear of patients and challenging environment as the most cause of psychological work-related health risk factors.

Table 16

Dental nurses' knowledge about the psychological work-related health risk factors (n=50)

Knowledge about psychological risk factors	No.	%
***Health risk factors**		
Emotional exhaustion	14	28.0
Depression	11	22.0
Depersonalization	26	52.0
***Causes of health risk factors**		
Anesthetization of patients	18	36.0
Excessive workload	25	50.0
Pain and fear of patients	13	26.0
Challenging environment	10	20.0

*Responses are not mutually exclusive.

Table (17) shows that, 90% of dentists choose emotional exhaustion as the most psychological work-related health risk factors affecting them while only 20% and 10% of dentists respectively choose depression and depersonalization. Related to causes of psychological work-related health risk factors, the table reveals that, 85.3% of dentists choose excessive workload, 58.7% of dentists choose anesthetization of patients while 61.3% of dentists choose the pain and fear of patients, also 80% of dentists choose challenging environment.

Table 17

Dentists' knowledge about the psychological work-related health risk factors (n=150)

Knowledge about psychological risk factors	No.	%
***Health risk factors**		
Emotional exhaustion	135	90.0
Depression	30	20.0
Depersonalization	15	10.0
***Causes of health risk factors**		
Anesthetization of patients	88	58.7
Excessive workload	128	85.3
Pain and fear of patients	92	61.3
Challenging environment	120	80.0

*Responses are not mutually exclusive.

Figure (20) depicts that, 80% of dental nurses' knowledge is unsatisfactory about different types of work-related risk factors while 20% of dental nurses' knowledge is satisfactory about the different types of work related risk factors.

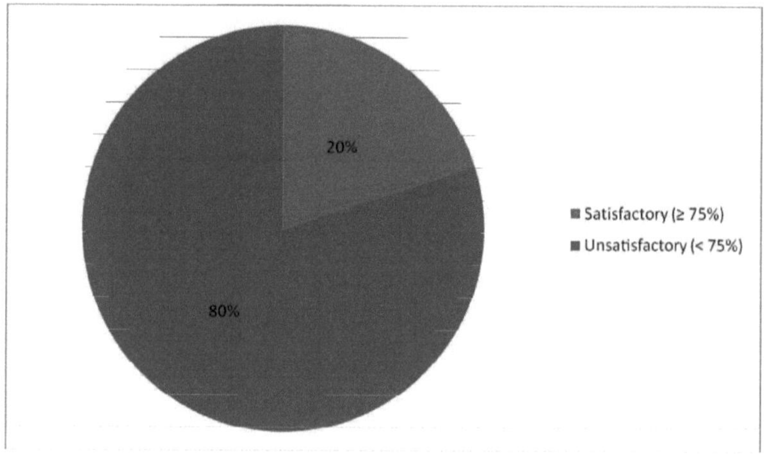

Figure 20. *Dental nurses' knowledge about work related health risk factors (n=50)*

Figure (21) indicates that, (47%) of dentists' knowledge is satisfactory and (34%) of dentists' knowledge is unsatisfactory while only (19%) of dentists' knowledge is good towards the different types of work related risk factors.

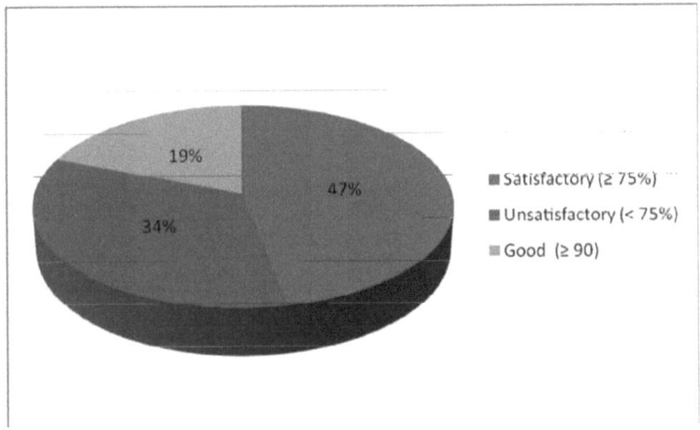

Figure 21. *Dentists' knowledge about work related health risk factors (n=150)*

Part III: Preventive health care measures applied by dental nurses and dentists.

Table (18) reveals that, only 10% of dental nurses do hand wash before patient contact and 40% of dental nurses do hand wash after patient contact while 50% of them do hand wash after touching of contaminated object. Regarding the wearing of PPE, the table shows that, 100% of dental nurses wear powdered latex gloves and 40% wear surgical mask while no one of dental nurses wears eye protector. In addition to, no one of dental nurses' change their uniform if contaminated.

Table 18

Distribution of observed practices among dental nurses regarding preventive measures for biological risk factors (n=50)

Biological preventive measures	Done		Not Done	
***Hand washing**	**No.**	**%**	**No.**	**%**
Before patient contact	5	10.0	45	90.0
Between each patient	10	20.0	40	80.0
After patient contact	20	40.0	30	60.0
After touching of contaminated objects	25	50.0	25	50.0
Use of alcohol rub	10	20.0	40	80.0
***Using of PPE**				
Powdered latex gloves	50	100	0	0.0
Plastic gloves.	35	70.0	15	30.0
Gloves are discarded after each patient	50	100	0	0.0
Wearing of surgical mask	20	40.0	30	60.0
Wearing eye protector	0	0.0	50	100
Wearing head cover	0	0.0	50	100
Uniforms changed daily	50	100	0	0.0
Uniforms changed if contaminated	0	0.0	50	100

*Responses are not mutually exclusive.

Table (19) reveals that, 23.3% of dentists do hand wash before patient contact and only 13.3% of them do hand washing after patient contact while 66.6% of dentists use an alcohol rub. Regarding wearing of PPE, the table shows that, 100% of dentists wear powdered latex gloves and 86.6% of dentists wear surgical mask while only 10% of dentists wear eye protector. In addition to, no one of dentists change uniform if contaminated.

Table 19

Distribution of observed practices among dentists regarding preventive measures for biological risk factors (n=150)

Biological preventive measures	Done		Not Done	
***Hand washing**	**No.**	**%**	**No.**	**%**
Before patient contact	35	23.3	115	76.6
Between each patient	30	20.0	120	80.0
After patient contact	20	13.3	130	86.6
After touching of contaminated objects	15	10.0	135	90.0
Use of alcohol rub	100	66.6	50	33.3
***Using of PPE**				
Powdered latex gloves	150	100	0	0.0
Plastic gloves.	110	73.3	40	26.6
Gloves are discarded after each patient	150	100	0	0.0
Wearing of surgical mask	130	86.6	20	13.3
Wearing eye protector	15	10	135	90
Wearing head cover	30	20	120	80
Uniforms changed daily	150	100	0	0.0
Uniforms changed if contaminated	0	0.0	150	100

*Responses are not mutually exclusive.

Table (20) indicates that, 100% of dental nurses work in good ventilated space, use safe solutions and high power suction also, 100% of dental nurses' use tightly closed capsule of mercury and store in sealed containers while no one of dental nurses wear hypoallergenic non-latex gloves and that indicate to the risk of latex allergy among dental nurses.

Table 20

Distribution of observed practices among dental nurses regarding preventive measures for chemical risk factors (n=50)

*Chemical preventive measures	Done		Not Done	
	No.	%	No.	%
Working in good ventilated space	50	100	0	0.0
Wearing of hypoallergenic gloves	0	0.0	50	100
Use safe solutions	50	100	0	0.0
Use high power suction	50	100	0	0.0
Use mercury tightly closed capsule	50	100	0	0.0
Stored mercury in sealed containers	50	100	0	0.0

*Responses are not mutually exclusive.

Table (21) indicates that, 100% of dentists work in good ventilated space, use safe solutions and high power suction also, 100% of dentists use tightly closed capsule of mercury and store in sealed containers while only 30% of dentists wear latex free gloves.

<u>Table 21</u>

Distribution of observed practices among dentists regarding preventive measures for chemical risk factors (n=150)

*Chemical preventive measures	Done		Not Done	
	No.	%	No.	%
Working in good ventilated space	150	100	0	0.0
Wearing of latex free gloves	45	30.0	105	70.0
Use safe solutions	150	100	0	0.0
Use high power suction	150	100	0	0.0
Use mercury tightly closed capsule	150	100	0	0.0
Stored mercury in sealed containers	150	100	0	0.0

*Responses are not mutually exclusive.

Table (22) clarifies that, 100% of dental nurses recap the needles after injection, 100% of them use sharp containers and disposal of waste materials properly also 100% of dental nurses store sharp instrument properly while no one of dental nurses wears neither face shield nor eye goggle during their contact with patients. Also, no one of dental nurses wears apron when exposed to x-ray radiation.

<u>Table 22</u>

Distribution of observed practices among dental nurses in relation to preventive measures for physical risk factors (n=50)

*Physical preventive measures	Done		Not Done	
	No.	%	No.	%
No recapping of needles	0	0.0	50	100
Use of sharp containers	50	100	0	0.0
Proper disposal of waste materials	50	100	0	0.0
Proper storage of sharp instruments	50	100	0	0.0
Wearing of aprons for ionizing radiation	0	0.0	50	100
Use of audible signals on machines when exposure is ended	50	100	0	0.0
Wearing of face shields	0	0.0	50	100
Wearing of eye goggles	0	0.0	50	100

*Responses are not mutually exclusive.

Table (23) clarifies that, 100% of dentists recap the needle after injection, 100% of them use sharp containers and disposal of waste materials properly also 100% of dentists store sharp instrument properly while no one of dentists wears neither face shield nor ear plugs during their contact with patients while only 10% of dentists wear eye goggles. Also, no one of dentists wears apron when exposed to x-ray radiation.

Table 23

Distribution of observed practices among dentists in relation to preventive measures for physical risk factors (n=150)

*Physical preventive measures	Done		Not Done	
	No.	%	No.	%
No recapping of needles	0	0.0	150	100
Use of sharp containers	150	100	0	0.0
Proper disposal of waste materials	150	100	0	0.0
Proper storage of sharp instruments	150	100	0	0.0
Wearing of aprons for ionizing radiation	0	0.0	150	100
Use of audible signals on machines when exposure is ended	150	100	0	0.0
Wearing of face shields	0	0.0	150	100
Wearing of eye goggles	15	10.0	135	90.0
Wearing of earplugs	0	0.0	150	100

*Responses are not mutually exclusive.

Table (24) reveals that, 50% of dental nurses can change their position frequently and can reach to instrument easily while no one of dental nurses can schedule patients in an effort to reduce the effects that result from mechanical health risk factors and no one of dental nurses can adjust their work station.

Table 24

Distribution of observed practices among dental nurses in relation to preventive measures for mechanical risk factors (n=50)

*Mechanical preventive measures	Done		Not Done	
	No.	%	No.	%
Changing position frequently	25	50	25	50
Scheduling patients	0	0	50	100
Adjust work station	0	0	50	100
Reaching instrument easily	50	100	0	0

*Responses are not mutually exclusive.

Table (25) reveals that, no one of dentists uses ergonomically designed chairs nor magnification devices during their dealing with patients. Related to changing of working position, no one of dentists can change their position during their work. Also, no one of dentists can schedule patients in an effort to reduce the effects that result from mechanical health risk factors while 100% of dentists use automatic and ultrasonic instrument and can adjust their work station. In addition, 50% of dentists can reach instrument easily.

Table 25

Distribution of observed practices among dentists regarding preventive measures for mechanical risk factors (n=150)

*Mechanical preventive measures	Done		Not Done	
	No.	%	No.	%
Use ergonomically designed chairs	0	0	150	100
Use automatic and ultrasonic instrument	150	100	0	0
Use magnification devices	0	0	150	100
Changing position frequently	0	0	150	100
Scheduling patients	0	0	150	100
Adjust work station	150	100	0	0
Reaching instrument easily	75	50	75	50

*Responses are not mutually exclusive.

Table (26) indicates that, 50% of nurses can plan ahead for emergency situations and feel appreciate from their supervisors, also their work is appreciated from their supervisor while only 20% of dental nurses can reassure their patients and only 30% modify their environment.

Table 26

Distribution of observed practices among dental nurses regarding preventive measures for psychological risk factors (n=50)

*Psychological preventive measures	Done		Not Done	
	No.	%	No.	%
Modification of environment	15	30	35	70
Reassuring of patients	10	20	40	80
Plan ahead for emergency	25	50	25	50
Appreciated work from supervisors	25	50	25	50

*Responses are not mutually exclusive.

Table (27) indicates that, 100% of dentists can plan ahead for emergency situations while only 10% of dentists feel the appreciation from their supervisors and modify their environment, and 50% of dentists can reassure their patients.

Table 27

Distribution of observed practices among dentists regarding preventive measures for psychological risk factors (n=150)

*Psychological preventive measures	Done		Not Done	
	No.	%	No.	%
Modification of environment	15	10	135	90
Reassuring of patients	75	50	75	50
Plan ahead for emergency	150	100	0	0
Appreciated work from supervisors	15	10	135	90

*Responses are not mutually exclusive.

Figure (22) indicates that, 75% of dental nurses' practices of preventive measures are unsatisfactory while only 25% of dental nurses' practices of preventive measures are satisfactory.

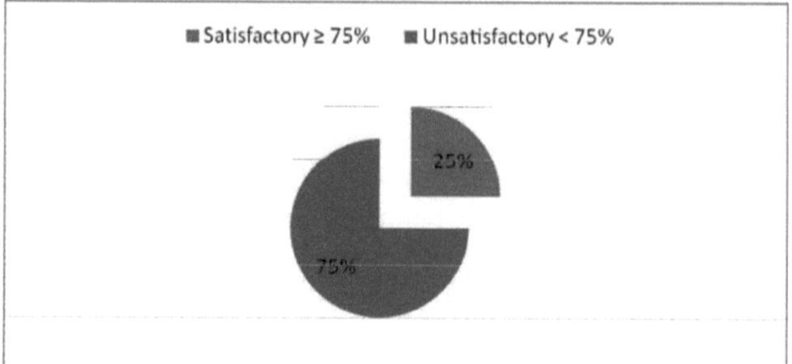

Figure 22. *Total scores of preventive measures application among dental nurses (n=50)*

Figure (23) indicates that, (60%) of dentists' practices of preventive measures are unsatisfactory while (34%) of dentists' practices of preventive measures are satisfactory. Only, (6%) of the dentists' practices of preventive measures are good.

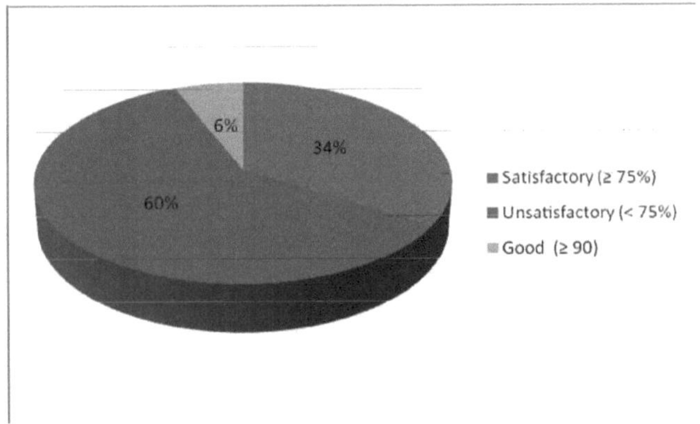

Figure 23. *Total scores of preventive measures application among dentists (n=150)*

Dental nurses' total knowledge and observed practices regarding work-related health risk factors are displayed in Figure (24) 80% of dental nurses' knowledge regarding work-related health risk factors is unsatisfactory and 75% of the dental nurses' observed practices of preventive measures are unsatisfactory.

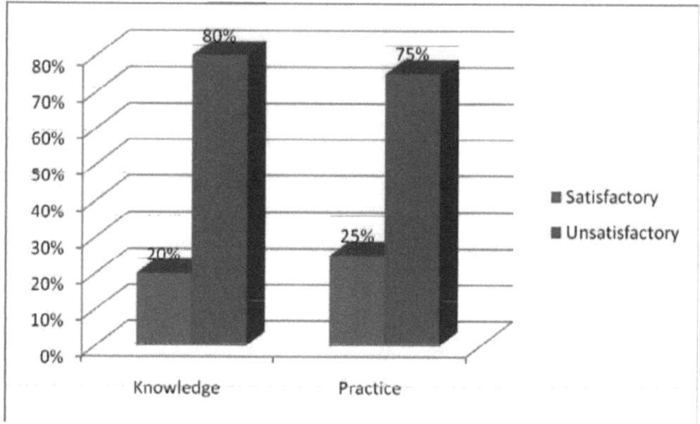

Figure 24. *Total knowledge and observed practices of dental nurses working in the dental clinic (n=50)*

Dentists' total knowledge and observed practices regarding to work-related health risk factors are displayed in Figure (25) and can be noticed that, 47% of dentists' knowledge regarding work-related health risk factors is satisfactory while only 19% of dentists' knowledge is good. Also, (34%) of dentists' observed practice is satisfactory while 60% dentists' observed practice is unsatisfactory and only 6% of dentists' observed practice is good.

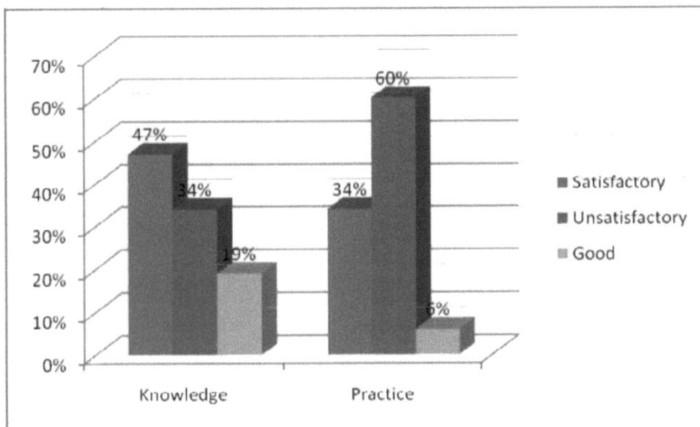

Figure 25.*Total knowledge and observed practices of dentists working in the dental clinic (n=150).*

Part IV: The relations between work-related health risk factors and preventive healthcare measures among dental nurses and dentists.

Table (28) indicates that, there is a statistically significant difference between years of experience and dental nurses' total practice scores.

<u>Table 28</u>

<u>*Total dental nurses' knowledge and practices score regarding their years of work experience (n=50)*</u>

Variables	Years of work experience				F	P
	<1 year	1-5 years	6-10years	> 10years		
	Mean ± SD	Mean ± SD	Mean ± SD	Mean ± SD		
Total knowledge scores	18.71±5.8	19.56±4.3	19.90±3.9	21.44±4.2	0.563	0.642
Total practice scores	44±1.6	43.39±2.4	42.18±2.6	45.33±3	2.735	0.045*

Table (29) clarifies that, no statistically significant correlation between dental nurses' knowledge towards different types of work-related health risk factors and dental nurses' observed practices towards preventive measures.

<u>Table 29</u>

Correlation between dental nurses' knowledge and observed practices (n=50)

Variables	Total Practice Scores	
	r value	p value
Total Knowledge Scores	-0.086	0.551

Table (30) reveals that, there is a statistically significant negative correlation between the incidence of chemical health risk factors and application of chemical preventive measures.

Table 30

Correlation between work related health risk factors and applied preventive measures among dental nurses (n=50)

Workplace health risk factors	Applied preventive measures	R	P
Chemical health risk factors	Chemical preventive measures	-0.274	0.045*
Physical health risk factors	Physical preventive measures	-0.011	0.940
Mechanical health risk factors	Mechanical preventive measures	0.134	0.355
Psychological health risk factors	Psychological preventive measures	0.047	0.746

* Correlation is significant at the level of < 0.05

Table (31) indicates that, there is a statistically significant difference between marital status and total knowledge scores while no statistically significant difference was found between marital status and total practice scores among dentists.

Table 31

Total dentists' knowledge and practice scores regarding their marital status (n=150)

	Marital status			
	Single	Married		
Variables	Mean ± SD	Mean ± SD	**T**	**P**
Total knowledge scores	25±3.1	25±3.9	6.581	0.011*
Total practice scores	49±10.5	50±12.2	0.473	0.637

* Correlation is significant at the level of < 0.05

Table (32) clarifies that, there is no statistically significant correlation found between dentists' knowledge towards different types of work-related health risk factors and dentists' observed practices towards preventive measures.

Table 32

Correlation between dentists' knowledge scores and dentists' observed practices (n=150)

Variables	Total Practice Scores	
	r value	**p** value
Total Knowledge Scores	-0.009	0.910

* Correlation is significant at the level of < 0.05 ** Correlation is highly significant at the level of < 0.01

Table (33) indicates that, there is a statistically significant negative correlation between the incidences of mechanical health risk factors and application of mechanical preventive measures. The table also indicates that, there is no statistically significant correlation between chemical, physical and psychological work risk factors and preventive measures.

<u>Table 33</u>

Correlation between work related health risk factors and applied preventive measures among dentists (n=150)

Workplace health risk factors	Applied preventive measures	R	P
Chemical health risk factors	Chemical preventive measures	0.082	0.320
Physical health risk factors	Physical preventive measures	-0.130	0.112
Mechanical health risk factors	Mechanical preventive measures	-0.177	0.030*
Psychological health risk factors	Psychological preventive measures	-0.009	0.915

* Correlation is significant at the level of < 0.05

Table (34) indicates that, there is a highly statistically significant difference between physical, psychological health risk factors where dentists have slightly higher mean scores than dental nurses.

<u>Table 34</u>

Correlation between work related health risk factors among dental nurses (n=50) and dentists (n=150)

Work place health risk factors		Dental nurses	Dentists	T	P
Chemical risk factors	Mean± SD	0.66± 0.55	0.53± 0.51	0.14	0.141
Physical risk factors	Mean± SD	1.28±1.03	1.84±0.895	3.728	0.000**
Mechanical risk factors	Mean± SD	3.06±1.2	3.31±0.833	1.596	0.112
Psychological risk factors	Mean± SD	1.72±1.03	2.20±1.02	2.903	0.004**

** Correlation is highly significant at the level of < 0.01

Table (35) indicates that, there is a highly statistically significant difference between biological, chemical, physical, mechanical preventive health care measures and type of job as dentists have higher mean scores than dental nurses. However, there is a highly statistically significant difference between psychological preventive health care measures and job where dental nurses have higher mean scores than dentists.

<u>Table 35</u>

<u>*Correlation between application of health care preventive measures among dental nurses (n=50) and dentists (n=150)*</u>

Applied preventive measures		Dental nurses	Dentists	T	P
Biological preventive measures	Mean ± SD	12±1.8	15.7±0.66	6.296	0.000**
Chemical preventive measures	Mean ± SD	10±0.0	10.6±0.91	7.991	0.000**
Physical preventive measures	Mean ± SD	12±0.0	12.2 ±0.60	4.069	0.000**
Mechanical preventive measures	Mean ± SD	1.0±1.01	6.0±0.00	5.300	0.000**
Psychological preventive measures	Mean ± SD	8.56±1.6	5.40±0.41	7.899	0.000**

** Correlation is highly significant at the level of < 0.01

CHAPTER V

Discussion

Dental nurses and dentists were constantly exposed to specific number of work-related health risk factors that categorized as, physical, mechanical, chemical, biological and psychological as PEI, low back pain, latex allergy, Hepatitis B and stressful situation. Awareness regarding this work-related health risk factors and implementation of preventive health care measures could provide a safe work environment for all dental nurses and dentists (Gamphir *et al*, 2011). So this study aimed at assessing the work-related health risk factors and application of preventive health care measures among fifty dental nurses and one hundred and fifty dentists were the subjects of this study.

The present study had investigated the various factors associated with work-related health risk factors as well as related preventive measures applied by both dental nurses and dentists in the dental clinics. Dental nurses were unique characteristics in dental clinics, especially in Cairo-University Hospitals. The current study results revealed that the most of dental nurses and more than two thirds of dentists were females also more than one third of studied dental nurses aged from 35-40 years while more than two thirds of studied dentists aged from 25-29 years.

This finding was in agreement with Saleh, (2010) a study done in dental health care centers at Cairo governorate on 50 dental nurses and 200 dentists who found that, the study sample of dental nurses was all females and the most of the dentists were females and one third of the dental nurses aged from 35 and above and more than two thirds of dentists aged from 20-29. From the investigator point of view, regarding to dental nurses these results might be related to see females working as nurses than males with the exclusion of some specialties and their age represented the majority of nursing staff in

Egypt while for studied dentists these results might be related to that dentists' females approved to participate in the study more than males and their age represented a category of studied dentists were selected in the study.

Also, the results of this study clarified that, two thirds of studied dental nurses and the majority of studied dentists were married. Related to level of education, the majority of studied dental nurses had secondary school nursing education while the majority of dentists had master degree. For the years of work experience, two thirds of dental nurses and the half of dentists had less than six years of work experience. These results agreed with Saleh, (2010) who found that, the majority of dental nurses and dentists were married and all of dental nurses had secondary school nursing education while the majority of dentists had bachelor degree and related to years of experience the majority of dental nurses and dentists had less than five years of work experience.

Regarding work services rendered for the studied dental nurses and dentists, the results of this study indicated that one third of them were doing a medical check-up with a frequency of more than one year and the minority of them had done medical check-up either less than 6 months or one year. Concerning training of studied dental nurses and dentists, more than two thirds of them got continuous training courses while less than half of them got pre-employment training courses. In relation to safety of the work environment, the majority of studied dental nurses and dentists were vaccinated against hepatitis B virus.

The results of this study agreed with the study done by Saleh, (2010) who found that, one third of dental nurses while more than half of dentists got training courses. Also, more than half of dental nurses and the majority of dentists get vaccination against hepatitis B virus in their workplace. My point of view that the presence of an infection control unit in Faculty of Oral and Dental Medicine offered a vaccine against Hepatitis B Virus and continuous training regarding work health risk factors and preventive health care measures for all dental nurses and dentists.

Related to biological work-related health risk factors prevailing among dental nurses and dentists, the results of this study revealed that, no one of them complained about any blood borne diseases as Hepatitis B, or Hepatitis C and HIV. The results of this study agreed with Ammon *et al*, (2010) who studied 215 dentists and 108 dental nurses in Berlin and found that only one of studied dental nurses and the minority of dentists had serological evidence of previous HBV and no one of dental nurses while the minority of dentists had serological evidence of HCV infection, also two third of dental nurses and dentists immunized against Hepatitis B.

Related to studied dental nurses, the results of this study agreed with the study done by Awooda & Homeda, (2014) on 127 dental nurses worked at dental teaching hospitals in Khartoum state and found that, the minority of dental nurses were positive to at least one marker of hepatitis markers, while the results of this study contradicted by the results of Awooda & Homeda, (2014) and found that the minority of dental nurses were vaccinated against Hepatitis B. Regarding to studied dentists, the results of this study agreed also to a study done by Isfahan, (2012) among dentists in India and found that, no one of studied dentists complained about any blood borne diseases as Hepatitis B, or Hepatitis C and HIV. From the investigator point of view, these results might be related to proper application of biological preventive measures by studied dental nurses and dentists as wore of latex gloves, wore of protective clothes and used of sharp containers and proper disposal of waste materials. Also, the majority of them were immunized against HBV.

Concerning the chemical work-related health risk factors, the results of this study revealed that, slightly less than two thirds of dental nurses and more than half of dentists complained of latex allergies. These results agreed with Yusoff *et al,* (2013) a study done in Malaysia and found that, more than one quarter of dental nurses and dentists complained from latex allergies. Related to studied dentists, the results were supported by Gupta *et al,* (2012) in their study in private dental clinics in India on 113 dentists and found that, one quarter of dentists complained of latex allergies.

Regarding latex allergies, the results of this study also agreed with the study done by Al-Ali *et al,* (2012) in the Emirates among 844 dentists, Agrawal, Bahatt, Singh, Chaudhary, & Asawa, (2010) among dentists in India and Isfahan, (2012) and found that one fifth of dentists complained of latex allergies. Related to the investigator point of view, the high prevalence of latex allergy among studied dental nurses and dentists might be related to all of them wore powdered latex gloves, and depended on an extensive number of literature reviews powdered latex gloves was considered the major cause of latex allergy. In addition, the results of this study revealed that, no one of dental nurses and dentists complained from mercury toxicity as a type of chemical work-related health risk factors and that might be related to proper application of chemical preventive measures by studied dental nurses and dentists as appropriate storage of mercury in tightly closed and sealed containers, used on high power suction and worked in good ventilation clinic.

In relation to physical work-related health risk factors, the results of this study revealed that, more than one third of dental nurses and more than two thirds of dentists complained of eye injury. Regarding to studied dental nurses, the results of this study contradicted with the study done by Albdour & Othman, (2010) in Jordan which indicated that, minority of dental nurses complained from eye injury while the results of the current study supported by the results of study done in Jordan which indicated that, two thirds of dentists complained from eye injury.

The results of this study contradicted with the results of the study done by Gupta et al, (2012) and study results of Isfahan, (2012) who found that the minority of dentists complained of eye injury. From the investigator point of view, the results of this study might be related to improper application of physical preventive measures by studied dental nurses and dentists as no one of them wore eye goggle during their contact with patients and according to an extensive number of literature reviews the use of eye goggle was an appropriate method of protection from eye injury.

Another type of physical work-related health risk factors was percutaneous exposure incident, the results of the study revealed that one third of dental nurses and all of dentists complained from percutaneous exposure incident. This results were in the same line with a study done by Shimoji, Ishihama, Yamada, & Okayama, (2010) on dental nurses and dentists at a single educational center in Japan who found that two third of dental nurses and more than half of dentists complained of injury from sharp instrument. For studied dental nurses, this result was in agreement with a study done by British Association of Dental Nurses, (BADN, 2014) which done in a Governorate hospital in England among dental nurses and reported that, more than half of dental nurses complained from percutaneous exposure incident.

Also, the results of this study agreed with Prabhu et al, (2014) who studied 102 dental nurses in India and found that, one third of dental nurses complained from needle stick injury in the past 6 months. While for studied dentists, the results were supported by Gupta et al, (2012) and Isfahan, (2012) and revealed that the majority of dentists complained from needle stick injury and injury from sharp instrument. Related to the investigator point of view, the results of this study might be related to recapping of anesthesia needles after injection to patients, unavailability of needle stick protector in dental clinics and injury from contaminated sharp instrument particularly when dental nurses cleaning it. Another type of physical work-related was hearing difficulties; the result of this study found that minority of dental nurses and dentists complained of hearing difficulties. For studied dentists, the results of this study agreed to a study done by AL-Ali *et al,* (2012), Isfahan, (2012) and Gupta *et al,* (2012) who found that the minority of dentists complained of hearing problems. From the investigator point of view, these results might be related to noise induced from dental equipment.

Regarding mechanical work-related health risk factors, results of this study revealed that, more than two third of dental nurses and most dentists complained from low back pain. Also half of dental nurses and the majority of dentists complained of neck pain, while less than one third of dental nurses and more than two thirds of dentists complained of wrist pain. In addition, more than one third of dental nurses and the majority of dentists complained of shoulder pain. For studied dental nurses, the results of this study were supported by Abdul Samat, Shafie, Yaccob, & Yussof, (2011) who studied dental personnel in Malaysia and found that, more than half of dental nurses complained of low back pain. Also results of this study agreed with Morse, Bruneau, & Dussetschleger, (2010) who studied dental health care workers in Italy and found that were less than two third of dental nurses complained of shoulder and neck pain. Moreover, Yasobant & Rajkumar, (2014) who studied dental health care workers in India, found that more than half of dental nurses complained from work-related musculoskeletal disorders.

Related to studied dentists, the results of this study agreed to a study done by Kaul, Shilpa, & Sanjy, (2015) among 150 dentists in the city of Bengaluru in Bengal and found that, more than half of dentists complained of low back pain, slightly less than half of dentists complained from neck pain, more than one quarter of dentists complained of shoulder pain while the minority of dentists complained from wrist pain. The results also, was supported by Al-Ali *et al,* (2012) who found that, more than two thirds of dentists complained of musculoskeletal problems and it was the most common occupational problem among the studied dentists. Also, Gupta *et al,* (2012) found that more than one third of dentists complained of musculoskeletal problems.

In the same line with this result, Isfahan, (2012) found that more than one third of dentists complained of one or more musculoskeletal problems. Also Feng, Liang, Wang, Andersen, & Szeto, (2014) who studied dentists in China, supported the results of this study and revealed that the majority of dentists complained of shoulder pain, more than two thirds of dentists complained of neck pain and more than half of dentists complained from wrist pain. The results of this study were supported by the study done by Botha, Chikte, Barrie, & Esterheuizen, (2014) on 338 dentists in South Africa and found that, the majority of dentists complained from neck pain, more than two thirds of dental nurses complained of shoulder pain and more than two thirds of dentists complained of low back pain. From the investigator point of view, the causes of high prevalence of mechanical work-related risk factors differed from dental nurses and dentists related to differences in the nature their work. For studied dental nurses the following causes of mechanical work-related risk factors might be related to harmful working postures, inadequate handling of equipment, improper workplace design, inadequate work organization and inappropriate application of mechanical preventive measures. For studied dentists the following causes of mechanical work-related risk factors might be related to awkward posture followed by improper workplace ergonomics, prolonged static posture, prolonged sitting in poorly designed chairs and repetitive movements.

Related to psychological work-related health risk factors, the results of this study revealed that, the majority of dental nurses and all of dentists complained of emotional exhaustion while less than one third of dental nurses and more than half of dentists complained of depression. Also, less than one third of dental nurses and dentists complained of depersonalization. For studied dental nurses, the results of this study contradicted with Peterson, Demerouti, Bergstorm, Asberg, & Nygren, (2011) a study done among 170 dental nurses in Sweden and found that, the minority of dental nurses complained of emotional exhaustion and more than one third of dental nurses complained of depersonalization.

Regarding studied dentists, the results were supported by Gupta *et al,* (2012) found that more than one third of dentists complained from job-related stress. In the same direction with this result, Isfahan, (2012) found that more than one third of dentists complained of emotional exhaustion. From the investigator point of view, the causes of psychological work-related risk factors differed from dental nurses and dentists related to differences in the nature of their work. For studied dental nurses the following causes of psychological work-related risk factors might be related to workload, low job control, job dissatisfaction, monotonous work and low support from coworkers and management. While the causes for studied dentists might be related to low autonomy, work overload, and inappropriate relation between power and responsibility and their teaching role in addition to their clinical role.

Related to studied dental nurses' and dentists' knowledge regarding the biological work-related health risk factors and its causes, the results of this study revealed that one third of dental nurses and the most of dentists chose Hepatitis B as a common health risk factor. Regarding causes of biological work-related health risk factors, more than one third of dental nurses and all of dentists chose cuts by contaminated dental equipment and direct contact with blood and body fluids. These results agreed with Saleh, (2010) who found that, two thirds of dental nurses and dentists chose anesthesia injection was more risk factors for transmission of blood borne diseases and more than half of dental nurses chose direct contact with saliva considered as a risk factor for transmission of blood borne diseases.

Regarding to studied dentists, the results of this study agreed to a study done by Mashlah, (2012) on 107 dentists in Syria about awareness of dentists regarding occupational health hazards and found that, more than half of dentists reported Hepatitis B and the majority of dentist reported HIV as the most biological health risk factors that might affect them and from the investigator point of view, the studied dental nurses and dentists had sufficient knowledge about different types of biological health risk factors and its causes that might be gained from continuous training that received from the infection control unit that present in their workplace.

Related to knowledge of the chemical work-related health risk factors and its causes, the results of this study revealed that, less than two thirds of dental nurses and all of dentists chose latex allergy and more than one third of dental nurses and dentists chose mercury toxicity as the most common type that might affect them. Regarding causes of chemical work-related health risk factors, less than two thirds of dental nurses and the majority of dentists chose not to wear non latex gloves as the major cause of chemical health risk factors.

Concerning to studied dentists, the results of this study agreed with the study done by Mashlah, (2012) who found that more than half of dentists chose mercury toxicity was the chemical health risk factor affecting them. The results of this study revealed from the investigator point of view that the studied dental nurses had insufficient knowledge regarding the chemical health risk factors and its causes and that might be related to that they didn't receive any training courses about it from the unit of infection control. While the studied dentists had sufficient knowledge regarding the chemical health risk factors and its causes that might be gained from self learning training courses.

Related to knowledge of the physical work-related health risk factors and its causes, the results of this study revealed that two thirds of dental nurses and all of dentists chose percutaneous exposure incident as the most risk factor affecting them. In relation to causes of physical work-related health risk factors, more than one third of dental nurses and the most of dentists chose not to use of sharp containers as the main cause of physical health risk factors. For studied dental nurses, the results of this study contradicted the study done by Prabhu *et al,* (2014) who found that the minority of dental nurses chose not to use sharp containers as the main cause of needle stick injury. Regarding the studied dental nurses and dentists, they had sufficient knowledge about the physical health risk factors and its causes that might be gained from continuous training that received from the infection control unit that presented in their workplace.

Related to knowledge of the mechanical work-related health risk factors and its causes, the results of this study revealed that more than two thirds of dental nurses and all of dentists chose low back pain and shoulder pain as a mechanical health risk factor that affected them. In relation to causes of mechanical work related health risk factors, more than two third of dental nurses and the majority of dentists chose incorrect sitting posture while the majority of dentists chose the repetitive use of manual instrument as the most causes of mechanical work-related health risk factors.

Concerning to studied dentists, the results of this study agreed with the study done by Mashlah, (2012) who found that more than two thirds of dentists chose low back pain as the mechanical health risk factor that might affect them. In relation to causes of mechanical work related health risk factors, the majority of dentists chose incorrect sitting posture and repetitive use of manual instrument as the most causes of mechanical work-related health risk factors. The studied dental nurses and dentists had sufficient knowledge about mechanical health risk factors and its causes as a result of their work experience and their previous or current complaining of this health risk factor.

Related to knowledge of the psychological work-related health risk factors and its causes, the results of this study clarified that one third of dental nurses and the minority of dentists chose depersonalization and more than one quarter of dental nurses and the majority of dentists chose emotional exhaustion as health risk factors that affect them. Regarding causes of psychological work-related health risk factors that, half of dental nurses and the majority of dentists chose excessive workload while more than one third of dental nurses and more than half of dentists chose anesthetization of patients as the most cause of psychological work-related health risk factors and this explained that the studied dental nurses had inadequate knowledge about psychological work-related health risk factors and its causes that might be related to they didn't receive any training courses about this health risk factors and its causes while the studied dentists had adequate knowledge as a result of their work experience and their previous or current complaining of this health risk factor.

The results of this study revealed that, the majority of dental nurses' knowledge were unsatisfactory while less than one quarter of dental nurses' knowledge was satisfactory towards the different types of work-related health risk factors and its causes. Regarding to dentists' knowledge, more than one third of dentists' knowledge was satisfactory and one third of dentists' knowledge was unsatisfactory while less than one quarter of dentists' knowledge was good towards the different types of work-related health risk factors and its causes. From the investigator point of view, the dentists were more knowledgeable than dental nurses and that might be related to dentists had higher education than dental nurses and depended on self learning training courses rather than dental nurses.

Regarding biological preventive measures applied by studied dental nurses and dentists, the results of the study found that more than one quarter of them were doing hand washing before patient contact. Regarding to wearing of PPE, the results showed that, all of dental nurses and dentists wore powdered latex gloves and protective clothes while no one of dental nurses and the minority of dentists wore eye protector. These results were in the same direction with a study done by Saleh, (2010) who found that, less than one quarter of dental nurses and dentists were doing hand washing before patient contact, the majority of them wore latex gloves and protective coat, also no one of dental nurses and the minority of dentists wore eye protector. From the investigator point of view, these results might be related to that studied dental nurses and dentists applied these steps from biological preventive measures might be related to fear of punishment from the infection control unit according to the investigator point of view.

Regarding studied dental nurses, the result of this study revealed that, no one of dental nurses wore eye protector, these results contradicted with the study done by Albdour & Othman, (2010) and found that, one third of dental nurses wore eye protection routinely.

For studied dentists, the results of this study agreed to a study done by Mutters, Hagele, Hagenfeld, Helwing, & Frank, (2014) among dentists in a university hospital in England and found that, one third of dentists washed their hands before patient contact and all of dentists wore gloves during their contact with patients while all dentists wore eye protector. Regarding to eye protection, these results might be related to the unit of infection control didn't supply the dental clinics with eye protectors for both dental nurses and dentists while for studied dentists who wore eye protector, they bought it at its expense didn't offer for them and that increase the prevalence of eye injury among dental nurses and dentists.

Regarding chemical preventive measures, all of dental nurses and dentists used tightly closed capsule of mercury and stored it in sealed containers while no one of dental nurses and slightly less than one third of dentists wore latex free gloves. For studied dentists, the results of this study agreed with the study done by Gupta *et al,* (2012) who found that more than half of dentists used tightly closed capsule of mercury and stored in sealed containers. From the investigator point of view, the results of this study might be related to that the Faculty of Oral and Dental Medicine supplied all dental clinics in the faculty by this type of mercury and was avoided the usage of the other types of mercury to prevent all dental nurses and dentists from the incidence of mercury toxicity while the faculty didn't supply the dental clinics with latex free gloves and for studied dentists who wore latex free gloves, they bought it at its expense didn't offer for them and that increase the prevalence of contact dermatitis among dental nurses and dentists.

Regarding physical preventive measures, the results of this study revealed that, all of studied dental nurses and dentists used sharp containers and recapped the needle after injection. No one of dental nurses or dentists wore apron when exposed to x-rays. According to wearing of protective measures, no one of dental nurses or dentists wore a face shield. For studied dental nurses, the results of this study contradicted the study done by Saleh, (2010) who found that all studied dental nurses didn't use sharp containers for disposal of sharps and needles after injection while the same study agreed with the results of this study regarding to dentists and found that all of dentists used sharp containers and recapped the needle after patient injection.

These results agreed with the study done by Prabhu *et al,* (2014) and found that the minority of dental nurses used needle safety measures. The results of this study might be related to that studied dental nurses and dentists applied these steps from physical preventive measures might be related to fear of punishment from the infection control unit according to the investigator point of view. On the other side, the infection control unit didn't supply dental clinics with the other physical preventive measures as face shield, apron and needle stick protector and that led to prevail of physical health risk factors among dental nurses and dentists.

The results of this study clarified the dental nurses' practices regarding application of mechanical preventive measures that half of dental nurses could change their position frequently while no one of dental nurses could schedule patients in an effort to reduce the effects that result from mechanical health risk factors. Related to dentists' practices regarding the application of mechanical preventive measures, no one of dentists could change their position during their work. Also, no one of dentists could schedule patients in an effort to reduce the effects that result from mechanical health risk factors.

From the investigator point of view, the results revealed the inappropriate practices of dental nurses and dentists regarding application of mechanical preventive measures and that might be related to work overload in the dental clinics, they couldn't able to change their working position frequently and the unavailability of mechanical preventive measures devices as ergonomically designed chairs nor magnification devices in the different dental clinics and that led to prevail of mechanical health risk factors among dental nurses and dentists.

The results of this study revealed the dental nurses' practices regarding the application of psychological preventive measures that half of dental nurses could plan ahead for emergency situations; also half of dental nurses were felt appreciation from their supervisor while less than quarter of dental nurses could reassure their patients. Regarding to dentists' practices for the application of psychological preventive measures, all of dentists could plan ahead during emergency situations because there were triage clinics for emergency situations and every dentist trained with this situation while the minority of dentists could modify their work environment. Also, the minority of dentists their work could be appreciated from supervisors. These results revealed the inappropriate practices of dental nurses and dentists regarding application of psychological preventive measures and that might be related to lack of knowledge about stress management and relaxation techniques and that might lead to prevail of psychological health risk factors.

The results of this study clarified that, more than two third of dental nurses' practices regarding preventive measures were unsatisfactory while a quarter of dental nurses' practices regarding preventive measures were satisfactory. Regarding the dentists' practices of preventive measures, the results of this study revealed that, less than two third of dentists' practices in relation to preventive measures were also unsatisfactory, one third of the dentists' practices of preventive measures were satisfactory while the minority of dentists' practices of preventive measures were good. From the investigator point of view, the majority of dental nurses and dentists couldn't apply proper practices regarding preventive health care measures and that lead to prevailing of different work-related health risk factors among dental nurses and dentists.

The results of this study revealed that, there was statistically significant difference between years of experience and total practice scores among dental nurses. These results were inconsistent with the study done by Saleh, (2010) who found that, there was no significant difference between the practices of dental nurses and years of experience. The results of this study showed that there wasn't a statistically significant difference between dental nurses' knowledge towards different types of work-related health risk factors versus dental nurses' observed practice towards preventive measures.

These results agreed with a study done by Saleh, (2010) and found that there was also no significant relation between knowledge of dental nurses and their practice while the results of this study revealed that, there was a statistically significant negative correlation between the incidence of chemical health risk factors and application of chemical preventive measures and that might be related to high prevalence of chemical health risk factors especially latex allergy among dental nurses and inappropriate application of chemical preventive measures as all dental nurses wore latex gloves.

The results of this study illustrated that, there was a statistically significant difference between marital status and total knowledge scores while no statistically significant difference was found between marital status total practice scores among dentists. These results agreed to a study done by Saleh, (2010) who found that, there was no significant difference between marital status total practice scores among dentists while there was statistically significant difference between marital status and total knowledge score.

Moreover, there wasn't a statistically significant correlation between dentists' knowledge towards different types of work-related health risk factors versus dentists' observed practice towards preventive measures. These results corresponded to a study done by Saleh, (2010) who found that there was no substantial relation between knowledge of dentists and their patterns. The results of this study showed also, there was a statistically significant negative correlation between mechanical health risk factors and application of mechanical preventive measures and that might be related to the high prevalence of mechanical health risk factors among dentists and inappropriate application of mechanical preventive measures.

Likewise, the results of this study clarified that, there was a highly statistically significant difference between physical work-related health risk factors, psychological work-related health risk factors and type of job where dentists had higher mean scores than dental nurses. From to the investigator point of view these results might be related to that studied dentists exposed to physical work-related health risk factors and psychological work-related health risk factors more than the studied dental nurses.

Related to application of preventive health care measures, the results of this study showed that, there was a highly statistically significant difference between biological, chemical, physical, mechanical preventive health care measures and job where dentists had higher mean scores than dental nurses and that explained from the investigator point of view that dentists could able to apply biological, chemical, physical and mechanical preventive health care measures more than dental nurses. However, there was highly statistically significant difference between psychological preventive health care measures and job as dental nurses had higher mean scores than dentists and that might be related

dental nurses could able to apply psychological preventive measures more than dentists.

CHAPTER VI

Summary, Conclusion and Recommendation

Summary

In carrying out their professional work, dental nurses and dentists were exposed to a number of work-related health risk factors. These factors cause the appearance of various ailments specific to the profession, which developed and intensified with years. In many cases, they resulted in diseases and disease complexes, some of which were regarded as work-related illnesses. Theses health risk factors categorized as physical, mechanical, chemical, biological and psychological. Therefore, dental nurses and dentists should be aware of preventive health care measures as appropriate sterilization or other high-level disinfection utilities, hepatitis B vaccination and continuing education about how to ergonomically use the instruments and effective time management (Fasunloro & Owotade, 2012). The more proper application of preventive health care measures, the least exposure to the work-related health risk factors.

Therefore, the aim of the study was to assess the work-related health risk factors among dental nurses and dentists and the preventive health care measures applied among dental nurses and dentists.

<u>Research Questions</u>

To fulfill aim of this study, the following research questions were formulated:

Q.1.   What are the work-related health-risk factors that prevailing among dental nurses and dentists?

Q.2.   What are preventive health care measures that are applied by dental nurses and dentists?

Subjects and methods

A descriptive cross-sectional research design was adopted in this study. A sample of convenience, 50 dental nurses and 150 dentists working in different dental clinics at the Faculty of Oral and Dental Medicine, Cairo University were included in the study. The study was conducted over 6 consecutive months.

To achieve the aim and answer the research questions following tools was formulated:

1- Socio-demographic questionnaire.

2- Work-related health risk factors questionnaire.

3- Structured observational checklist.

The main findings of the current study were as follows:

Regarding the socio-demographic characteristics of dental nurses and dentists, the most of dental nurses (98%) and more than two thirds of dentists were females (68.6%). More than one third of studied dental nurses aged from 35-40 years (36%) while more than two thirds of studied dentists aged from 25-29 years (69.3%). Also, two thirds (62%) of studied dental nurses and more than two third (68.6%) of studied dentists were married. In relation to level of education, the majority (90%) of studied dental nurses had a secondary school nursing education, while more than half (56%) of dentists had master degree. For the years of work experience, less than half (46%) of dental nurses and half (50%) of dentists had less than six years of work experience.

125

Concerning to biological work-related health risk factors prevailing among dental nurses and dentists, no one of them complained about any of blood borne diseases as hepatitis B, or hepatitis C or HIV and that was related to proper application of biological preventive measures by studied dental nurses and dentists as all (100%) of dental nurses and dentists wore latex gloves protective clothes and used sharp containers and proper disposal of waste materials.

Related to chemical work-related health risk factors about two thirds (62%) of dental nurses and slightly more than half (53%) of dentists complained from latex allergies. Also, no one of dental nurses and dentists complained from mercury toxicity and all (100%) of them used chemical preventive measures appropriately and stored of mercury in tightly closed and sealed containers, used on high power suction and worked in a good ventilation clinic while all (100%) of them wore powdered latex gloves that cause latex allergy.

Concerning physical work-related health risk factors, more than one third (40%) of dental nurses and more than two thirds (68.7%) of dentists complained from eye injury and that might be related to improper application of physical preventive measures by studied dental nurses and dentists as no one of them wore eye goggle during their contact with patients. Also, one third of dental nurses (34%) and all (100%) of dentists complained from percutaneous exposure incident and that included, complain from needle stick injury as (100%) of them recapped needles of anesthesia after injection to patients and unavailability of needle stick protector in dental clinics. In addition, the minority of dental nurses and dentists complained of hearing difficulties as a result from noise induced from dental equipment and that no one of them wore earplugs.

Regarding mechanical work-related health risk factors, three quarters (76%) of dental nurses and 93.3% of dentists complained of low back pain also, half (50%) of dental nurses and majority (86.7%) of dentists complained of neck pain. While less than one third (30%) of dental nurses and more than two thirds (69.3%) of dentists complained from wrist pain, more than one third (40%) of dental nurses and the majority (82%) of dentists complained of shoulder pain. The causes of high prevalence of mechanical work-related risk factors were related to inappropriate application of mechanical preventive measures. For studied dental nurses, half (50%) of them changed their position frequently and no one of them adjusted work station and scheduled patients. For studied dentists, no one of dentists used ergonomically designed chairs nor magnification devices during their dealing with patients. In Relation to changing of working position, no one of dentists could change their position while working.

In relation to psychological work-related health risk factors, the results of this study revealed that, majority (82%) of dental nurses and all (100%) of dentists complained of emotional exhaustion while less than one third (28%) of dental nurses and more than half (54%) of dentists complained of depression. Also, less than one third (28%) of dental nurses and dentists complained of depersonalization and that might be related to improper following of psychological preventive measures. In relation to studied dental nurses, half (50%) of them could plan ahead for emergency situations and felt appreciated from their supervisors. For studied dentists, all (100%) of dentists could plan ahead for emergency situations while the minority (10%) of dentists felt the appreciation from their supervisors.

The results of the study presented that there was a statistically significant correlation between years of experience and total practice scores among dental nurses. No statistically significant correlation was found between dental nurses' knowledge towards different types of work-related health risk factors and dental nurses' observed practice towards preventive measures while there was statistically significant negative correlation between the incidence of chemical health risk factors and application of chemical preventive measures among dental nurses.

Also results of this study illustrated that there was a statistically significant correlation between marital status and total knowledge scores among dentists. Moreover, no statistically significant correlation was found between dentists' knowledge about different types of work-related health risk factors and their observed practices towards preventive measures. Also, there was a statistically significant negative correlation between the incidences of mechanical health risk factors and application of mechanical preventive measures among dentists.

Conclusion:

Based on the result of the current study; it can be concluded that:

There was a gap between dental nurses' knowledge and dentists' knowledge regarding work-related health risk factors and its causes. While, both of dental nurses and dentists had inadequate practices related to physical, mechanical and psychological preventive health care measures. There was a statistically significant negative correlation between the incidence of chemical health risk factors and application of chemical preventive measures among dental nurses. Also, there was a statistically significant negative correlation between the incidence of mechanical health risk factors and application of mechanical preventive measures among dentists.

<u>Recommendations</u>

Based on the study results, the following recommendations were suggested:-

- Offer educational programs and upgrading courses armed with evidence based guidelines based on dental nurses' and dentists' needs to improve their knowledge and practice related to work-related health risk factors and preventive measures.

- Specific training program should be designed for dental staff about proper use of preventive health care measures related to the dental field.

- Dentistry work-related health risk factors and its preventive measures should be integrated into the nursing curriculums.

- Further research is needed to evaluate the current study variables on a larger sample to generalize the study results.

References

Abdul Samat, R. J., Shafie, M. N.,Yaccob, N. A., & Yussof, A. E. (2011). Prevalence and associated factors of back pain among dental personnel in North-Eastern State of Malaysia. International Journal of Collaborative Research on Internal Medicine and Public Health; 3, 576-586.

Adel, H. K., & Mostafa, H. T. (2012). A Study of Occupational health problems among a group of dental laboratory technicians in Alexandria city. Available at:(http//www.researchgate.net).

Agrawal, A. N., Bahatt, N. D., Singh, K. F., Chaudhary, H. M., & Asawa, K. S. (2010). Prevalence of allergy to latex gloves among dental professionals in Udaipur, Rajasthan, India. Oral Health Preventive Dental Journal; 8, 345-350.

Al-Ali, B. N., Khalid, H. M., & Raghad, K. N. (2012). Occupational health problems of dentists in the United Arab Emirates. International Dental Journal; 52-56. Available at: (http//www. onlinelibrary.wiley.com/journal).

Albadour, M. J., & Othman, E. R. (2010). Eye Safety in Dentistry. Pakistan Oral and Dental Journal; 30, 8-13.

Al-Eisa, N.J. (2011). Effects of pelvic asymmetry and low back pain on trunk kinematics during sitting: a comparison with standing. Spine; 5, 135–143.

American Dental Association Journal (ADA, 2012). Safety Issues. Available at:(www.dentalclinicmanual.com/docs/SafetyIssues).

Ammar, M. H., Samer, S. D., & Sharif, A.S. (2009). A study of Exposure Dentists in Damascus to some occupational risks. Damascus University for Health Sciences Journal; 25, 30-40.

Ammon, A. N., Reichart, P. O., Pauli, G. K., & Petersen, L. S. (2010). Hepatitis B and C among Berlin dental personnel: incidence, risk factors, and effectiveness of barrier prevention measures. Epidemiological infection journal; 125, 407-413.

Anyel, S. G., & Scully, C. H. (2011). Occupational hazards in Dentistry. Occupational health hazards in current dental profession; 3, 57-64.

Awooda, E. D., & Homeda, Y. O. (2014). Hepatitis B Virus serological test among nurses working in Dental teaching hospitals in Khartoum State. International Journal of Nursing Didactics;4.Availableat:http//www.innovativejournal.in/ijnd/index.php/ijnd/article/view/ 2.

Babji, P. L., Samadi, F. V., Jaiswal, J. W., & Bansal, A. M. (2011). Occupational hazards among dentists. Journal of International Dental and Medical Research; 4, 87-93.

Barrientos, M. K., & Driscoll, D. B. (2012). Selected occupational risk factors. Comparative Quantification of Health Risks Article. Available at : http//www.who.net.

Bell, D.T. (2010). Occupational risk of human immunodeficiency virus infection in health care workers: an overview. American Journal of Medicine; 102(5B), 9-15.

Botha, P. N., Chikte, U. C., Barrie, R. K., & Esterheuizen, T. P. (2014). Self-reported musculoskeletal pain among dentists in South-Africa. South-Africa Dental Journal; 69, 208-213.

Brand, D. T., & Chalmar, H. E. (2011). General health of dentists. Litetrature review. Dental and Maxillofacial Journal; 9, 10-20.

Branson, B. E., Bray, K. W., Gadbury, C. S., Holt, L. O., & Keselyak, N. A. (2008). Ergonomics and Injury in the Dental Office. The Academy of Dental Therapeutics Stomatology. Available at: (http// www.ineedce.com).

Brar, R. J., & Karar, H. E. (2011). Occupational hazards in current dental profession. The Open Occupational of Health and Safety Journal; 57-64. Available at: (http://creativecommons.org/licenses/by-nc/3.0/).

British Association of Dental Nurses (BADN, 2014). Over half of dental nurses have had a needle stick injury article; 217, 50-54.

Buchta, W. J., & Russi, M. T. (2012). Guidance for occupational health services in medical centers (2nd ed); pp 12.California.

Center for Disease Control and Prevention (CDC, 2010a). Transmission of hepatitis B and C viruses in outpatient settings-New York, Oklahoma and Nebraska, 2000-2002. MMWR; 52(38): 901-6.

CDC. (2010b). Recommended infection-control practices for dentistry. MMWR; 42(8): 1-13.

Charpin, D. T., & Vervolet, D. K. (2011). Occupational hazards in current dental profession. The Open Occupational of Health and Safety Journal; 9, 57-64. Available at: (http://creativecommons.org/licenses/by-nc/3.0/).

Cheng, H. N., Haung, C. M., & Yen, A. L. (2012). Needle Stick and Sharp Injuries. Plos One Journal; 1, 1-7.

Chikte, C. H., Naidoo, S. D., & Yengopal, V. A. (2011). Occupational Health Hazards in Current Dental Profession. The Open Occupational Health and Safety Journal; 3, 57-64. Available at: (http//www.benthamopen.com/toohsj/articles/V003/57TOOHSJ).

Dawson, O. S., Hallet, M. K., & Millinder, L. F. (2011). Occupational hazards in current dental profession. The Open Occupational of Health and Safety Journal; 5, 57-64. Available at: (http://creativecommons.org/licenses/by-nc/3.0/)

Depaola, L. H., Rodgers, P. U., & Hamann, C. H. (2010). General health of dentists. Baltic Dental and Maxillofacial Journal; 9, 10-20.

Dickinison, M.T. (2012). Sterilization and cross-infection control in the dental practice. Dental CPD journal;6,14-20.

Dunlap, J. F., & Stewart, J. T. (2011). Survey suggests less stress in group offices. Dent Econ 2011; 72, 46-54.

El-Eisa, E. N., Egan, D. L., Deluzio, K. P., & Wassersug, R. M. (2008). Ergonomics and Injury in the Dental Office. The Academy of Dental Therapeutics Stomatology. Available at: (http// www.ineedcc.com).

Ethridge, S. B., MacKellar, D. K., & Branson, B. D. (2005). Community Health Nursing, Roles of occupational Health Nurse, 5th edition. Lippincott Company, New York pp345-354.

Fariba, S. C., & Younai R. E. (2010). HealthCare-Associated Transmission of Hepatitis B &C Viruses in Dental Care. Clin Liver Dis; 14, 93-104.

Fasunloro, A. E., & Owotade, F. R. (2012). Occupational hazards among clinical dental staff. The Journal of Contemporary dental staff; 6, 1-10. Available at: (http://www.thejcdp.com).

Fauci, A. W., & Lane, H. N. (2010). Human immunodeficiency virus (HIV) disease: AIDS and related disorders. Harrison's Principles of Internal Medicine Journal ; 2, 1566-1618.

Feng, B. O., Liang, Q. L., Wang, Y. M., Andersen, L. L., Szeto, G. M. (2014). Prevalence of work-related musculoskeletal symptoms of the neck and upper extremity among dentists in China. BioMedical Journal; 4, 1136.

Feyer, A.T. (2012). Selected occupational risk factors. Comparative Quantification of Health Risks Article. Available at:(http//www.who.net).

Gamphir, R. K., Singh, G. M., Sharma, S. P., Brar, R. E., & Karar, H. S. (2011). Occupational hazards in current dental profession. The Open Occupational of Health and Safety Journal; 3, 57-64. Available at: (http://creativecommons.org/licenses/by-nc/3.0/).

Greenspan, J. K., & Scully, C. R. (2012). Critical Reviews in Oral Biology and Medicine. Dental Research Journal; 9, 794-800. Available at:(http://jdr.sagepub.com).

Greer, F.D. (2009). Latex Allergy among Health Care Workers .American Family Physician Journal;13,1414.

Gupta, M. H., Mehta, A. D., & Upadhyaya, N. T. (2012). Status of occupational hazards and its preventive among dental professionals. The Dental Research Journal;3, 446-451. Available at: (http://www.mui.ac.ir).

Hamann, C.A. (2012). Allergic Contact Dermatitis in Dental Professionals. American Dental Association Journal; 9, 185-194.

Houivs, M.O. (2010). Disinfection and sterilization: the duties and responsibilities of dentists and dental hygienists. International Dental Journal ; 42, 241-244.

Humphris, G.K. (2011). A review of burnout in dentists. Dental Update Journal; 25, 392-396.

Isfahan, J.M. (2012). Occupational hazards to dental staff. Dental Research Journal; 1, 2-7. Available at:(http://jdr.sagepub.com).

Jabbar, T.K. (2012). Musculoskeletal Disorders among Dentists in Saudi Arabia .Pakistan Oral and Dental Journal; 28, 135-144.Available at (www.podj.com.pk).

Kanski, M.D. (2010). Occupational hazards to dental staff. Journal of Contemporary dental staff; 9, 2-7.

Kaul, R. J., Shilpa, P. S., Sanjay, C. J. (2015). Musculoskeletal disorders and mental health related issues as occupational hazards among dental practitioners in the city of Bengaluru, randomized cross-sectional study. International Journal Medical and Dental Science; 4, 589-598.

Kedjarune, U. F., Leggat, P. V., & Smith, D. A. (2010). Occupational Health Problems in Modern Dentistry. The Industrial Health Journal; 45, 1-11.

Kilford, N.R. (2009). The National code of practice for the preparation of material safety data sheet journal; 5, 2).

Klein, R. B., Freeman, K. W., Taylor, P. L., & Stevens, E. U. (2005). Different roles of occupational health nurse. Lancet; 338,1539-42.

Kohn, W. G., Collins, A. S., Cleveland, J. L., Harte, J. A., Eklund, K. J., & Malvitz, D. M. (2010). Guidelines for infection-control in dental health care settings: a report originated in the national centre for chronic disease prevention and health promotion; 52, 1-61.

Lindbohm, M.H. (2014). Occupational exposure in dentistry and miscarriage. Occupational and Environment medicine; 2, 127-133.

Lyapena, M. F., Yaneva, A. I., Tzycova, M. H., & Garova, M. O. (2012). Allergic contact dermatitis from formaldehyde exposure. Journal of International Medical Association Belgaria); 18, 256-262.

Maillet, J. P., Millar, A. M., Burke, J. M., Maillet, M. A., Maillet, W. A., Neish, N. R. (2008). Effect of magnification loupes on dental hygiene student posture. Dental Education Journal; 72, 33–44.

Martin, M. B., & Naleway, C. H. (2011). Factors Contributing to mercury exposure in dentists. American Dental Association Journal; 3, 1502-11.

Mashlah, A.T. (2012). Study of information and sources of dentists about occupational hazards. Damascus University Journal for Medical Sciences; 1, 111-126.

Melchior, M. N., Evanof, B. J., & Chastang, J. A. (2012). Why are manual workers at high risk of upper limb disorders? The role of physical work factors in a random sample of workers in France (the Pays de la Loire study). (National Institute of Health Research); 11, 754–761.

Morse, T. D., Bruneau, H. I., Dussetschleger, J. K. (2010). Musculoskeletal Disorders of the neck and shoulder in the dental professions. PubMed Journal; 35. Available at: http// www. www.ncbi.nlm.nih.gov/pubmed.

Morse, T. R., Braunea, H. L, & Sanders, M. E. (2012). Musculoskeletal disorders of the neck and shoulder in dental hygienists and dental hygiene students. Dental Hygiene Journal; 1,10.

Mutters, N. T., Hagele, U. G., Hagenfeld, D. F., Helwing, E. N., & Frank, U. J. (2014). Compliance with infection control practices in a university hospital dental clinic. PubMed journal; 9. Available at: www.ncbi.nlm.nih.gov/pubmed.

National Institute of Occupational Safety and Health (NIOSH, 2012). Other Safety Issues : Eye Protection, Noise Control and Ventilation. The American Dental Association Journal; 45, 1-4.

National Library of Medicine. (2012). Prevention of health care measures. Available at : (http://www.wikipedia.com).

Neis, M. G., & Ewen, J. S. (2011). Community Health Nursing, Concepts and Practice, 5th edition. Lippincott Company, New York ; 66, 343-354.

Occupational Safety and Health Administration (OSHA, 2013). Guidance for occupational health services in medical centers (2nd ed); pp 12. Available at: (www.osha.gov).

Osborne, D. F., & Cruocher, R. T. (2011). Levels of burnout in general dental practitioners in the south-east of England. British Dental Journal ;177, 372-7.

Ostrem, C. H. (2011). Occupational hazards among dentists. Journal of International Dental and Medical Research; 4, 87-93. Available at:(http://www.ektodermaldisplazi.com/journal.htm).

Peterson, U. A., Demerouti, E. M., Bergstorm, G. B., Asberg, M. F., & Nygren, A. D. (2011). Work characteristics and sickness absence in burnout and non burnout groups, a study of Swedish health care workers. International journal of stress management; 15, 153-172.

Pollart, V.T. (2009). Latex Allergy among Medical Professionals. American Family Physician Journal; 3,1413.

Prabhu, A. L., Rao, A. P., Reedy, V. N., Sugumaran, K. F., Mohan, G. A., & Ahmed, S. J. (2014). Needle Safety Awareness among Dental Nurses. Workplace Health and Safety Journal; 62, 243-247.

Puriene, A.H. (2011). General health of dentists. Litetrature review. Stomatologija. Baltic Dental and Maxillofacial Journal; 9, 10-20.

Rada, R. K., & Johnson, L. F. (2011). Stress, burnout, anxiety and depression among dentists Journal of American Dental Association; 135, 788-94.

Reddy, M.C. (2009). Latex Allergy among Dental Health Care Workers .American Family Physician Journal;6,1415.

Regier, D. O., Row, D. W., & Narrow, E. D. (2011). Occupational hazards among dentists. Journal of International Dental and Medical Research; 4, 87-93. Available at:(http://www.ektodermaldisplazi.com/journal.htm).

Saleh, R.N. (2010). Knowledge, attitude and practice toward blood borne diseases (HBV, HCV& HIV) among dental health care worker thesis; 79-104.

Samaranayake, P.E. (2012). Re-emergence of tuberculosis and its variants: Implications for dentistry. International Dental Journal; 52, 330–336.

Sartolio, F. A., & Vercelli, S. J. (2012). Work-related musculoskeletal diseases in dental professionals. Prevalence and risk factors; 2, 165–169.

Shmoji, S. D., Ishihama, K. H., Yamada, H. N., & Okayama, M. L. (2010). Occupational safety among dental health care worker. Journal of Advances in Medical Education and Practice; 1, 41-47.

Shortdge, G. O., & McCauly, R. H. (2011). Community Health Nursing Caring in Action, second edition, Delmer Company, USA, pp 900-919.

Smith, D. S., Wilkinson, J. Y., Tadema, G. K., Evans, N. A., Jarrold, A. C., & Minson, E. N. (2010). Best Practices Guidelines for Occupational Safety and Health in Dental Therapy Practice; 72, 1-27.

Talaat, M. S., Kandeel, A. H., El-Shoubary, W. K., Boden S. C., Khairy, I. O., Oun, S. G., & Mahoney, F. J. (2010). Occupational exposure to needle stick injures and hepatitis B vaccination coverage among health care workers in Egypt. American Journal Inf Control; 31, 469-74.

Tosic, G.M. (2011). Occupational Hazards in Dentistry- Part One: Allergic reactions to dental restorative materials and latex sensetivity. Working and Living Environmental Protection; 2, 317-324.

Valachi, B. H., & Valachi, K. J. (2013). Musculoskeletal Disorders in Clinical Dentistry and Their Prevention. Orofacial research journal; 2, 106-114.

Valachi, B.H. (2010). Ergonomics and injury in the dental office. American Dental Association Journal(ADA); 3, 28-36.Available at (www.ineedce.com).

World Health Oraganization (WHO, 2010c). Hepatitis C. World health organization fact sheet. Available at: www.who.int/ media centre / fact sheets.

WHO. (2010b). Diseases of public health significance. Available at: www.world wide health.org.

WHO. (2011a). The Global Occupational Health Network; 12, 38-42. Available at: http://www.who.int /health info/boddaly/en/index.html.

WHO. (2011d). The Role of Occupational Health Nurse in Workplace Health Management; 2, 1-78. Available at: http:// www.who.int/occupational_health/regions/en/oeheurnursing.pdf

Yasobant, S. O., Rajkumar, P. N. (2014). Work-related Musculoskeletal Disorders Among Health Care Professionals: Across-sectional Assessment of risk factors in a tertiary Hospital, India. Indian Journal of Occupational and Environmental Medicine; 18, 75-81.

Yusoff, A. N., Murray, S. K., Abd Rahman, N. T., John, J. K., Mohammad, D. B, & Tin-oo, M. J. (2013). Self-Reported Latex Glove Allergy among Dental Personnel in Kelantan state, Malaysia. International Medical Journal; 20, 343-345.

عوامل الخطورة المرتبطة بالعمل والاجراءات الوقائية المتبعة بين ممرضات وأطباءالأسنان بكلية طب الفم والأسنان

مقدمة من الطالبة رسالة

مروة ممدوح شعبان
بكالريوس تمريض-جامعة القاهرة
معيدة بتمريض صحة المجتمع كلية التمريض-جامعة القاهرة

توطئة للحصول على درجة الماجستير فى علوم التمريض
(تمريض صحة المجتمع)

المشرفين

<table>
<tr><td>أ.د/ شيرين عزالدين طه</td><td>أ.د/ نجاة سعيد حبيب</td></tr>
<tr><td>أستاذ طب أسنان الصحة العامة كلية طب الفم</td><td>أستاذ تمريض صحة المجتمع كلية التمريض-</td></tr>
<tr><td>والأسنان- جامعة القاهرة</td><td>جامعة القاهرة</td></tr>
</table>

د/ إيمان محمود سيف النصر
مدرس تمريض صحة المجتمع كلية التمريض-
جامعة القاهرة

2015

عوامل الخطورة المرتبطة بالعمل والاجراءات الوقائية المتبعة بين ممرضات وأطباءالأسنان بكلية طب الفم والأسنان

رسالة مقدمة من الطالبة

مروة ممدوح شعبان

بكالريوس تمريض-جامعة القاهرة

معيدة بتمريض صحة المجتمع كلية التمريض-جامعة القاهرة

توطنة للحصول على درجة الماجستير فى علوم التمريض
(تمريض صحة المجتمع)

وقد تم مناقشة الرسالة والموافقة عليها

لجنة الحكم: التوقيع

أ.د/ نجاة سعيد حبيب
أستاذ بقسم تمريض صحة المجتمع- كلية التمريض- جامعة
القاهرة

أ.م.د/ وليد على محمد
أستاذ مساعد بقسم الصحة العامة- كلية طب الفم والأسنان-
جامعة القاهرة

أ.م.د/ جيهان مصطفى إسماعيل
أستاذ مساعد بقسم تمريض صحة المجتمع- كلية التمريض-
جامعة القاهرة

تاريخ الموافقة: /   /

الملخص العربى

المقدمة

يتعرض ممرضات الأسنان وأطباء الأسنان إلي عدد من عوامل المخاطر الصحية المرتبطة بعملهم وهذا أثناء القيام بعملهم بشكل مهني .و تتسبب هذه العوامل في ظهور العديد من الأمراض المرتبطة بالمهنة التي تتطور وتقوي عبر السنين . فانها في حالات عديدة تسبب امراض وتعقيدات مرضية والتي يعتبر بعضها من الأمراض المرتبطة بالعمل. وتصنف عوامل الخاطر الصحية إلي فيزيائى وميكانيكي وكيميائي وبيولوجي ونفسي. ولهذا ينبغي علي كلا من ممرضات وأطباء الأسنان أن يكونوا علي دراية بتدابير الرعاية الصحية الوقائية كالتعقيم المناسب وغيرها من مرافق التعقيم رفيعه المستوي والتطعيم ضد إلتهاب الكبد ب يجب ايضا استمرار التعلم والتعرف علي كيفية الاستخدام الهندسي للادوات وكيفية إداره الوقت بفعالية . فكلما كانت تطبيق تدابير الوقاية الصحية مناسبا كلما قل التعرض لعوامل المخاطر الصحية المرتبطة بالعمل.

الهدف من البحث:

تقييم لعوامل الخطورة المرتبطة بالعمل والاجراءات الوقائية المتبعة بين ممرضات وأطباءالأسنان بكلية طب الفم والأسنان .

تصميم البحث:

أستخدام البحث الوصفى للوصول لهدف الدراسة

عينة البحث :

تشمل عينة البحث على 50 من تمريض الأسنان و 150 من أطباء الأسنان الذين يعملون بالعيادات المتواجدة بكلية طب الفم والأسنان – جامعة القاهرة. وقد تم أختيارهم حسب المواصفات المحددة فى هذه الدراسة وهى: أن يكون من ممرضات وأطباء الأسنان بكلية طب الفم والأسنان جامعة القاهرة.

معايير الأستبعاد فى هذا البحث الصفات التالية :

1- ممرضات وطبيبات الأسنان الحوامل.

2- ممرضات وأطباء الأسنان الذين يعانون من الأمراض المزمنة.

3- ممرضات وأطباء الأسنان الذين تزيد أعمارهم عن 40 عاما.

مكان البحث:

تم تنفيذ هذا البحث فى العيادات المتواجدة بكلية طب الفم والأسنان جامعة القاهرة.

أدوات البحث:

أدوات البحث تشتمل على :-

1- إستمارة جمع بيانات ديموجرافية والتى تشتمل على:

أسئلة لمعرفة (السن، الجنس ، المؤهل الدراسي ، عدد سنوات العمل......... إلخ) لكل ممرضة أسنان وطبيب أسنان .

2- إستبيان لتقييم عوامل الخطورة المرتبطة بالعمل (تشتمل على أسئلة لتقييم معلومات ممرضات وأطباء الأسنان حول إدراكهم لهذه المخاطر وهل تعرضوا لأى أصابة بأى من هذه المخاطر).

3- أستمارة لملاحظة الأجراءات الوقائية المتبعة بين ممرضات وأطباء الأسنان (تشمل ملاحظة غسل اليدين وماهى أوقاتها المحددة و ارتداء القفاز وهل يتم أرتداء بقية الأدوات الشخصية الوقائية إلخ ....) وهذه الأستمارة قد قامت الباحثة بملئها وتجميع البيانات الخاصة بها.

تم أخذ الموافقات الرسمية لتنفيذ البحث من مجلس كلية التمريض و طب الفم والأسنان – جامعة القاهرة , وبعد شرح تفصيلى للهدف من الدراسة تم أخذ موافقة كتابية من كل تمريض وأطباء الأسنان الذين وافقوا على المشاركة فى هذه الدراسة.

النتائج الرئيسية للدراسة:-

أوضحت نتائج الدراسة ما يلى :-

- فيما يتعلق بالخصائص الديموغرافية للممرضات وأطباء الأسنان، ومعظم الممرضات (98)٪ وأكثر من ثلثي أطباء الأسنان من الإناث(68.6)٪ . بالنسبة لعمر ممرضات وأطباء الأسنان، أكثر من ثلث الممرضات الأسنان (36 ٪) تتراوح أعمارهم بين 40-35عاما في حين أن أكثر من ثلثي أطباء الأسنان (69.3%) الذين تتراوح أعمارهم بين 29-25سنة. وأيضا تقريبا ثلثي ممرضات (62%) و الغالبية من أطباء الأسنان (68.6%) متزوجون. وفيما يتعلق بالمستوى التعليمى فأن غالبية تمريض الأسنان حاصلين على دبلوم التمريض فى حين أن أكثر من نصف أطباء الأسنان حاصلين على درجة الماجستير.وبالنسبة الى سنوات الخبرة في العمل ، فأن ثلثي ممرضات الأسنان (46٪) ونصف 50% من أطباء الأسنان لديهم أقل من ست سنوات من الخبرة في العمل.

143

- فيما يتعلق بعوامل المخاطر الصحية البيولوجية المتعلقة بالعمل السائدة بين ممرضات الأسنان وأطباء الأسنان ,فلم يشتكي احدا منهم من اي من الأمراض النقولة عن طريق الدم كالإلتهاب الكبد الوبائي ب وسي او مرض نقص المناعة المكتسبة (الإيدز) ويرتبط هذا بالتطبيق المناسب للتدابير البيولوجية الوقائية عن طريق ممرضات الأسنان والاطباء ايضا . فكل 100% من ممرضات الأسنان وأطباء الأسنان يرتدون قفازات الاتكس ويرتدون الملابس الوقائية ويستخدمون الحاويات الحادة ويتخلصون من النفايات بطريقة سليمة .

- وفيما يتعلق بعوامل المخاطر الصحية الكيميائية المتعلقة بالعمل فأقل من ثلثي (62%) من ممرضات الأسنان وأكثر من النصف (53%) من أطباء الأسنان يعانون من حساسية الاتكس وأيضا لا أحد من ممرضات الأسنان وأطباء الأسنان قد أشتكي من تسمم الزئبق . ويرتبط هذا بالجميع 100% منهم يقومون بتطبيق التدابير الوقائية الصحية الكيميائية بالطريقة المناسبة . ويصبح الزئبق مخزن ومغلق بإحكام في حاويات محكمة الغلق ويقوموا ايضا بإستخدام المص بطاقة عالية ويعملون في عيادات ذات تهوية جيدة في حين 100% منهم يرتدون قفازات بمسحوق الاتكس التي تسبب حساسية الاتكس

- فيما يتعلق بعوامل المخاطر الصحية الفيزيائية المتعلقة بالعمل فإن أكثر من الثلث 40% من ممرضات الأسنان وأكثر من ثلثي (68.7%) من أطباء الأسنان يعانون من إصابات بالعين وربما يعود هذا إلي عدم التطبيق الجيد لتدابير الوقاية الفيزيائية من قبل ممرضات الأسنان وأطباء الأسنان . كما ان لا أحد منهم يرتدي حامي العين أثناء تعاملهم مع المرضي كما ان ثلث ممرضات الأسنان (34%) و 100% من أطباء الأسنان قد عانوا من حادثة تعرض عن طريق الجلد وهذا يشمل الشكوي من الوغز بالإبرة وهذا نتيجة لأن 100% منهم يقومون بإستعادة إبرة التخدير بعد حقن المرض بها و عدم إتاحة وجود حامي من وغز الإبرة في عيادات الأسنان بالإضافة إلي ان الأقلية من ممرضات الأسنان واطباء الأسنان يعانون من صعوبات في السمع كنتيجة للإزعاج الناتج من أدوات الأسنان وهذا أيضا مرتبط بعدم ارتداء أي منهم لسدادات الأذن .

- فيما يتعلق بعوامل المخاطر الصحية الميكانيكية المرتبطة بالعمل فإن أكثر من ثلثي (76%) من ممرضات الأسنان و الأغلبية (93.3 %) من أطباء الأسنان يعانون ايضا من الالام ف أسفل الظهر والنصف (50%) من ممرضات الأسنان والأغلبية (86.7%) من أطباء الأسنان يعانون من الالام في الرقبة في حين ان اقل من الثلث (30%) من ممرضات الأسنان وأكثر من ثلثي (69.3%) من الأطباء يعانون الالام في المعصم بلإضافة الي إن أكثر من الثلث (40 %) من ممرضات الأسنان والأغلبية (82%) من أطباء الأسنان يعانون من الالام في الكتف . ويعود السبب إلي الانتشار الكبير لعوامل المخاطر الميكانيكية المرتبطة بالعمل إلي التطبيق الغير مناسب لتدابير الوقاية الميكانيكية . فإن ممرضات الأسنان (50%) منهم يغيرون من وضعهم بشكل متكرر ولا أحد منهم يقوم بتعديل مكان العمل او المرضي الذين علي الانحة . اما بالنسبة إلي أطباء الأسنان فإن لا احد منهم يستخدم الكراسي المصممة هندسيا ولا أجهزة التكبير أثناء التعامل مع المرضي. فيما يتعلق بتغير وضع العمل فلا أحد من أطباء الأسنان يمكنه تغير وضعه أثناء عمله .

- فيما يتعلق بعوامل المخاطر الصحية النفسية المرتبطة بالعمل فقد أوضحت نتائج هذه الدراسة أن الأغلبية (82%) من ممرضات الأسنان والجميع (100%) من أطباء الأسنان قد عانوا من الإجهاد العاطفي بينما أقل من الثلث (28%) من ممرضات الأسنان وأطباء الأسنان قد عانوا من تبدد الشخصية وربما يعود هذا إلي الإتباع الغير جيد لتدابير الوقاية النفسية . فإن نصف ممرضات الأسنان (50%) منهم يمكنهم التخطيط مستقبلا لحالات الطوارئ ويشعرون بالتقدير من قبل مشرفيهم . اما بالنسبة إلي أطباء الأسنان فإن 100% منهم يمكنهم التخطيط مستقبلا لحالات الطوارئ بينما الأقلية (10%) منهم يشعرون بالتقدير من من قبل مشرفيهم .

- أوضحت نتائج هذه الدراسة أنه هناك إرتباط ذو دلالة إحصائية بين سنوات الخبرة ومعدل إجمالي الممارسة بين ممرضات الأسنان .ولم يكن هناك إرتباطا ذو دلالة إحصائية بين معلومات ممرضات الأسنان نحو الأنواع المختلفة لعوامل المخاطر الصحية المرتبطة بالعمل وملاحظة الممارسة تجاه تدابير الوقاية بينما هناك إرتباط سلبى ذو دلالة إحصائية بين حدوث المخاطر الصحية الكيمائية وتطبيق التدابير الوقائية الكيمائية.

- كما أوضحت أيضا نتائج هذه الدراسة أنه هناك إرتباط ذو دلالة إحصائية بين الحالة الإجتماعية ومعدل إجمالي المعلومات لدي أطباء الأسنان .علاوة علي ذلك لم يكن هناك أي إرتباط ذو دلالة إحصائية بين معلومات أطباء الأسنان عن الأنواع المختلفة لعوامل المخاطر الصحية المرتبطة بالعمل مقابل ملاحظة

الممارسة تجاه تدابير الوقاية وايضا هناك إرتباط سلبي ذو دلالة إحصائية بين حدوث المخاطر الصحية الميكانيكية وتطبيق التدابير الوقائية الميكانيكية

الخلاصة:

إستنادا إلى نتائج الدراسة الحالية يمكننا ان نستنتج انه :

- عوامل المخاطر الصحية المرتبطة بالعمل السائدة بين ممرضات الأسنان وأطباء الأسنان كانت كيميائية فيزيائية وميكانيكية وعوامل مخاطر نفسية .

- هناك فجوة بين معلومات ممرضات الأسنان وأطباء الأسنان تجاه عوامل المخاطر الصحية المرتبطة بالعمل ومسبباتها .

- ممرضات الأسنان وأطباء الأسنان لديهم ممارسات غير كافية تجاه تدابير الوقاية الصحية الفيزيائية والميكانيكية والنفسية .

- هناك إرتباط ذو دلالة إحصائية بين عوامل المخاطر الصحية الكيميائية وتدابير الوقائية الكيميائية المتبعة بين ممرضات الأسنان.

- هناك إرتباط ذو دلالة إحصائية بين عوامل المخاطر الصحية الميكانيكية وتدابير الوقائية الميكانيكية المتبعة بين أطباء الأسنان .

<u>التوصيات</u>

إستنادا إلى نتائج الدراسة فقد تم إقتراح التوصيات التالية :

- توفير بنامج تعليمي وتطوير الدورات المزودة بمبادئ توصية إلي أدلة من إحتياجات ممرضات الأسنان وأطباء الأسنان لتحسن معلوماتهم وممارستهم المتعلقة بعوامل المخاطر الصحية وتدابير الوقاية .

- برامج تدريبية تنفذ علي الوقاية وإستراتجيات المواجهة لعوامل المخاطر الصحية الميكانيكية والنفسية من خلال ممرضات الأسنان وأطباء الأسنان.

- تصميم برامج تدريبية خاصة لفريق عمل أطباء الأسنان عن الإستخدام المناسب لتدابير الوقاية الصحية المتعلقة بمجال طب الأسنان .

- يجب أن توحد في مناهج التمريض عوامل المخاطر الصحية المرتبطة بعمل طب الأسنان وتدابير الوقاية

- هناك حاجة إلي مزيد من البحوث لتقيم متغيرات الدراسة الحالية علي عينة أكبر لتعميم نتائج هذه الدراسة .

- يجب إصدار السياسات والإسترتيجيات لمكافحة عوامل المخاطر الصحية المرتبطة بالعمل في مجال عمل طب الأسنان .

- اللجوء إلي إختبار الفحص السمعي بشكل دوري للكشف المبكر لمشاكل السمع لممرضات الأسنان وأطباء الأسنان .

- رفع مسوي الوعي لممرضات الأسنان وأطباء الأسنان عن إتباع الطرق الناجحة للتحكم في الضغط ولتعامل افضل مع المريض وفي نهاية المطاف لممارسة أكثر نجاحا .

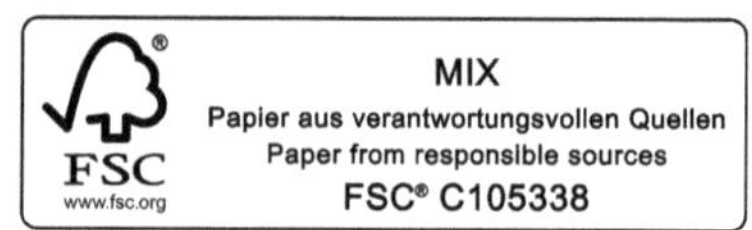

Printed by Books on Demand GmbH, Norderstedt / Germany